Routledge Revivals

I0129418

Some Early and Later Houses of Pity

From around the eleventh century until the Reformation, a close connection between the Church and hospitals was formed as they became a refuge for the ill, ostracised and poor. First published in 1926, John Morrison Hobson presents a fascinating survey of the hospitals and almshouses found throughout medieval England. Full of photographs and illustrations, Hobson surveys the almshouses by geographical location and provides a social and historical context for each. This practical and interesting study will be of use to students and academics with an interest in English hospitals and almshouses, their relationship to the Church, and English social history more generally.

Some Early and Later Houses of Pity

John Morrison Hobson

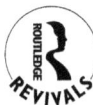

Routledge
Taylor & Francis Group

First published in 1926
by George Routledge and Sons Ltd

This edition first published in 2013 by Routledge
2 Park Square, Milton Park, Abingdon, Oxon, OX14 4RN

Simultaneously published in the USA and Canada
by Routledge
711 Third Avenue, New York, NY 10017

Routledge is an imprint of the Taylor & Francis Group, an informa business

© 1926 John Morrison Hobson

Publisher's Note
The publisher has gone to great lengths to ensure the quality of this reprint but points out that some imperfections in the original copies may be apparent.

Disclaimer
The publisher has made every effort to trace copyright holders and welcomes correspondence from those they have been unable to contact.

A Library of Congress record exists under LCCN: 26014907

ISBN 13: 978-0-415-82079-0 (hbk)
ISBN 13: 978-0-203-56237-6 (ebk)
ISBN 13: 978-0-415-82145-2 (pbk)

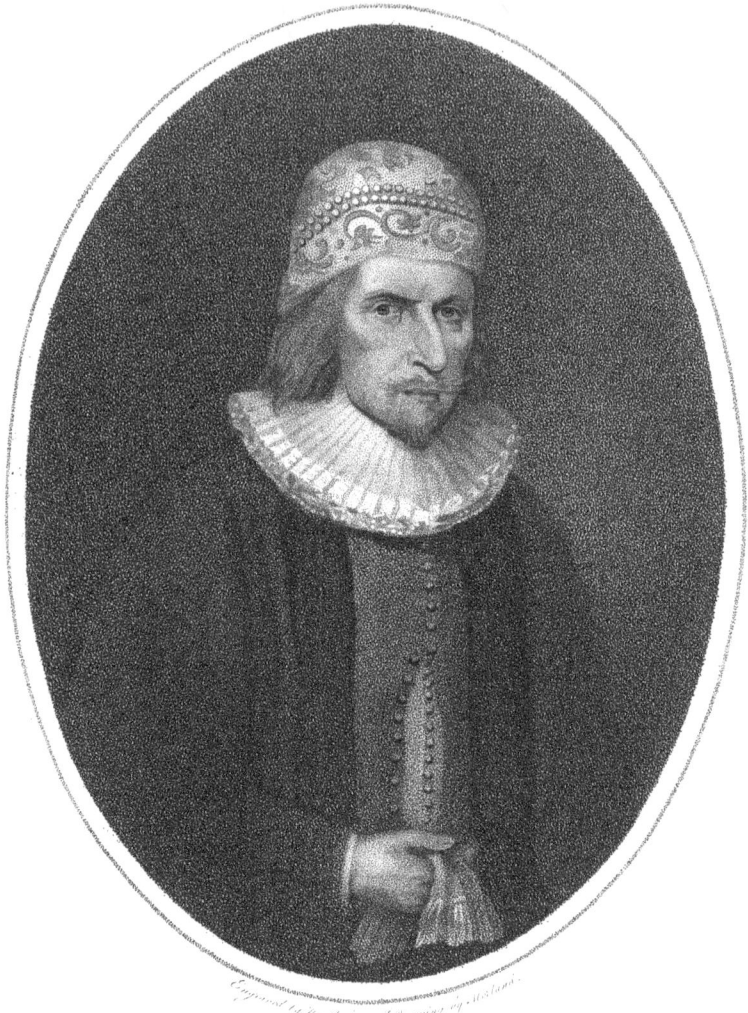

Engraved by Heath from a Drawing of Holland.

HUMFREDUS CHETHAM ARMIGER, *FUNDATOR*.

Natus 10 Julii 1580. *Obiit 12 Octobris 1653.*

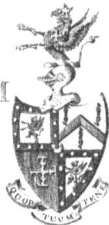

Ætatis 73.

A Tabula in Hospitio Chethamensi adservata.

SOME EARLY AND LATER HOUSES OF PITY

BY

JOHN MORRISON HOBSON, M.D., B.Sc.

Past President Croydon Nat. Hist. Soc., Member of Surrey Archæol. Soc.

Author of *The Arkwrights (an Elizabethan Romance); The Case for Whitgift's Hospital; The Book of the Wandle, etc.*

With numerous illustrations

LONDON

GEORGE ROUTLEDGE AND SONS, LTD.

BROADWAY HOUSE: 68-74, CARTER LANE, E.C.

1926

Printed in Great Britain by
MACKAYS LTD., CHATHAM

CONTENTS

LIST OF ILLUSTRATIONS

PLATES

vii

ILLUSTRATIONS IN THE TEXT

PREFACE

THIS partial survey of the ancient Houses of Pity in England had its origin in an intention to write more fully than had yet been done concerning Whitgift's famous hospital in Croydon. This beautiful old building had become familiar to me during my long residence in that town, through my friendship with Alfred Jones, B.A., its Warden, who died, aged 90, a few years ago.

But Whitgift's Hospital needed historic setting and thence grew the present attempt to give a **personality** to a selection from the ancient hospitals, schools, and almshouses which once have been or do still exist. Upon the foundation laid by Dugdale in his *Monasticon Anglicanum*, supplemented by his editors in 1830, have I built, as has Miss Clay in her book, to which frequent references will be found in my text. Other materials have been gathered from the Victoria County Histories; *Encyclopædia Britannica* (latest edition) and other works; by research into the archives of Whitgift's Hospital (chiefly extracted from Alfred Jones' Notes); and by my own observations. For further help in writing I wish to own my indebtedness to Mr. H. Keatley Moore, of Croydon, and Mr. Berwick Sayers and his staff at the Public Library in that town, who have shown me unfailing kindness; to Mr. Philip Palmer, Master of Abbot's Hospital; to Mr. J. W. Fielding, House Governor of Chetham's Hospital; to Mr. F. J. Causton, Master of St. Cross; to Prof. Claude Jenkins, of Lambeth Palace Library; to Prof. Sir A. E. Garrod; to Mr. C. G. Paget, of Croydon; to the late Mr. Streatfield, Warden of Whit-

gift's Hospital; and others whose names I may have
failed to mention.   In the case of illustrations, facilities
have been readily given by those in authority or on
the spot, and acknowledgments are recorded in their
proper places to those who have lent blocks, where my
own photographs did not avail.   I must, moreover,
record my especial indebtedness to the Governors of
Chetham's Hospital and Library for use of the valuable
plate from which the portrait of the founder in the
frontispiece has been taken, and to Messrs. G. Falkner
and Sons, of Manchester, for the loan of blocks illustrating the school.   These gentlemen have issued pictured
booklets which describe Chetham's Hospital more fully
than I have done.   It has been possible thus to impart
a pictorial interest to the northern counties which they
would otherwise have lacked.   Fortunately, Miss Clay
gives several illustrations of those parts.   The auto-
graph of Archbishop Abbot, shown on p. 141, is from a
small block lent by the Surrey Archæological Society.

Miss Clay's book should be read in conjunction with
this one.   She gives a multitude of word-pictures and
her work might be called a " general physiology " of
mediæval hospitals.   Those which I have produced,
mere outline sketches and meagre enough in many
cases through the scantiness of the data collected, are
an attempt at individual, concrete presentment.   Yet,
where possible, I have brought into view their relation-
ships with one another and with their environment.
My work is by no means exhaustive, as Miss Clay admits
of her own.   There must be a vast field in still existing
archives open for social historians to explore.   My
grouping of counties mainly follows the order of the
old Anglo-Saxon kingdoms.

We cannot afford to call ourselves " moderns," if it
implies a cutting off from the Past.   There is no " dead
past " ; it belongs to the Eternal, of which the Present

is but a phase.   The motives of our forefathers may look different from our own and their points of view were often widely divergent from ours.   Yet they likewise were living men, " modern " in their day, and at bottom much like ourselves.   In so far as their eyes were " single," they acted with sincerity, and our indebtedness to them is immeasurable.

J.M.H.

SOME EARLY AND LATER HOUSES OF PITY

CHAPTER I

INTRODUCTORY

Eftsoones unto an holy Hospitall,
That was foreby the way, she did him bring ;
In which seven Bead-men, that had vowed all
Their life to service of high heavens King,
Did spend their daies in doing godly thing.
Their gates to all were open evermore,
That by the wearie way were traveiling ;
And one sate wayting ever them before,
To call in commers-by that needy were and pore.

Spenser's *The Faerie Queene*, Book I.,
Canto X., 36.

ALMS, our own short word, comes from the prolonged and beautiful Greek eleēmosūnē (ἐλεημοσύνη), **Pity.**

Hospitals and almshouses are, indeed, abodes of pity, but they have come to have a present-day association somewhat different from the ideas of our forefathers. In fact, the word chosen in the title of this book seems apt, for *pity* is derived from the Latin *pietas*, and piety, as Christian thought conceived it in the middle ages, was inseparable from the motives which led to the building of hospitals in this country.

With the Romans, *hospes* stood both for a host and a guest. From a root *ghan* (Sanscrit *han*, to strike) came the Latin *hasta* a spear, *hostia* recompense, *hostis* an enemy or a foreigner and, strange as it may seem, the above word *hospes*. From this same common root were derived the English word *guest*, the Welsh *gwestai*, the Armoric *hostiz* and the Bohemian *host*, all having the same meaning, but also signifying a **Stranger.** How came it that applications apparently so diverse as " host," " guest " and " stranger " each originated in the unamiable notion of striking a blow ? Let us go back in imagination to primitive man. He is standing at the entrance to his cave or his hut. Presently a stranger approaches. " Surely he is an enemy," says he, " where is my spear ? " But as man advances towards civilisation, we see him acting on the safer assumption that the stranger has no evil intent and resolved to disarm him morally, if so be he has such motive, by offering him food, or at least salt and shelter. Hence it became the customary duty of the man of the tent to give these to the wayfarer, asking no questions. From this conception it is not difficult to go further and understand how to the Romans *hospes* signified both entertainer and entertained, *hospitalis* (hospitable) the quality which welcomed others, whether friends or strangers, and *hospitium* the place where guests were received. Hence the French acquired, in the one sense, the word *hospice*, where the helpless and the wayfarers were welcomed, as at Great St. Bernard, established in the eleventh century for the accommodation of those traversing that dangerous pass in the Alps, and, in another, *hospital* (now *hôpital*) for the treatment of the sick. The English, probably borrowing from the Continent,

applied from the beginning the word *inclusively* to places
for the temporary reception of travellers and pilgrims
and for the permanent care of the aged poor, the
" maimed, halt and blind," and for the cure of the sick.
The monasteries also had their *hospitium* for guests
or strangers, while their infirmary was not exclusively
for their own sick.

It is not true, as has been said, that hospitals were of
Christian origin, for they existed in remote times
amongst non-Christian peoples, although it does not
appear that they were invariably eleemosynary. Both
the ancient Egyptians and the Greeks were in the habit
of encouraging those who were afflicted to resort to the
temples, where the priests, who alone had any medical
knowledge, could treat them, and where their diseases
could be studied. In India, the Emperor Asoka
founded many hospitals for the sick as early as 260 B.C.,
that at Surat still existing. Although it does not
appear that the Romans employed any word exactly
corresponding to *hospital*, places of such a nature are
recorded in the time of the Emperor Hadrian (117 A.D.
–138) for wounded and sick soldiers. Galen, the
world-famous Greek physician (*c.* 130 A.D.–*c.* 205)
speaks of " Iatria " (Greek, *iatros*, a physician) in the
Roman Empire, where out-patients were treated for
small fees.

Coming to the Christian period after the cessation
of persecution, we hear of " Nosocomia " (Greek *nosos*,
a disease, and *comeo*, to tend) during the reign of
Constantine, these institutions being in connection with
the Church. From this onwards, we read of hospitals
by Basil at Cæsarea for lepers in 370, by Chrysostom

(*c.* 345–407) at Constantinople, by Augustine (354–430) at Hippo and of six hundred men specially chosen for their experience to tend the sick at Alexandria in 416.[1]

Benedict of Nursia in Umbria (*c.* 480–*c.* 544) was a good and great man. He founded many monasteries in Italy under a new rule. This, while giving first place to the " work of God," by which he meant religious services, by no means required the monks to spend the major part of the week-day in church. Much time was given to agriculture, study and education. In fact, the saying " laborare est orare," if not exactly attributable to the Benedictines, might be taken as one of their guiding principles. England was the seat of the first planting of the Benedictine rule out of Italy when, in 596, Augustine landed as missionary and regulator.[2]

Whatever we may think of the limitations of these men in England and notwithstanding later corruptions, we feel assured that *they*, at least, were in earnest and, with the world-wide appeal, which is a command, ever present in their minds, " I was a stranger and ye took me in," they were compelled to set up guest-houses for wayfarers and infirmaries for impotent folk in their monasteries, the forerunners of all and the type of many of the Houses of Pity later established in this land. The close connection between the Church and the hospitals, begun in these early centuries, was continued to a large extent, though not universally, up to the time of the great Dissolution.

---

[1] *Encyc. Brit.,* " Hospitals," by Sir Hy. Burdett.
[2] *Encyc. Brit.,* Rt. Rev. E. C. Butler, *Monasticon.*

Before passing, however, to our partial survey of the ancient hospitals of England, we must note that the Mahommedans did not neglect this kind of provision for members of their own religion. The Caliph Harūn al Rashid (763–809), of romantic memory, instituted a college and an asylum at every mosque. At Bagdad, there was an asylum for the insane open to all Moslem believers, besides a number of free infirmaries.[1] This liberal accommodation of the " Infidels " and their solicitude for the mentally afflicted is the more remarkable in that several centuries elapsed in Christian Europe before there was any thought of public care for the insane. This subject will be considered later but it may be observed here that the notion, perhaps adopted by the early Church from the Jews, that these unfortunates were possessed of devils which must be cast out, would probably account for this abstention and when, at length, places were provided for them, the motive of pity was a questionable factor.

Spenser's Canto X., from which the opening lines of this book are taken, gives us a good idea of a mediæval hospital, for he was much nearer those days than are we. Though, as Miss Clay says, the words "hospital," " bede-house " and "almshouse" were used indiscriminately, there is some difference.[2] The mediæval hospital was essentially a convent (*con*, together, *venio*, come), a religious house with a superior who was styled master most often, warden sometimes, and even occasionally keeper, and those who had devoted themselves to a religious life. All these had taken vows and, with

[1] Sir Hy. Burdett, *op. cit.*
[2] *Mediæval Hospitals of England*, Rotha Mary Clay, 1909.

sometimes lay brothers and sisters, constituted the staff. Many joined this convent as a refuge from the ills of life and, in theory at least, they were all poor, having given up their possessions. The mastership, on the other hand, if not originally so, became a living. Sir Julius Cæsar, in Elizabeth's time, not satisfied with the emoluments of his office, petitioned the Queen for the reversion of a mastership, and was eventually given that of St. Katharine by the Tower. We read, moreover, of the advowson frequently being conferred as if it were a valuable benefice. The pensioners were bedesmen or almsmen, not members of the conventual corporation, except in the case of a lazar-house. Lepers were outcasts from society because of their affliction and, doomed to spend the rest of their days in a hospital, took religious vows, even, according to Miss Clay, sometimes electing their master from among themselves. Even casual visitors and the sick had to take some part in the religious observance, while the permanent beneficiaries were obliged to join in them to a considerable extent, as at Ewelme.

It is not quite clear from the data which the present writer has collected, nor even from Miss Clay's book, what was the exact meaning of the term " poor men " frequently met with in the words of foundation, _i.e._. whether it _always_ implied almsmen or sometimes religious members of the staff. On the other hand, " brother " does not seem always to have meant one of the staff, for Miss Clay, quoting Eadmer, speaks of 100 poor brethren and sisters at St. John's, Canterbury. As we shall see, de Blois, so early as 1136, founded St. Cross " that the poor in Christ may there humbly and devoutly serve God." This suggests that the original thirteen beneficiaries were religious brethren. The term clings to the present inmates and was repeated by Whitgift, Abbot and Sutton.

CHAPTER II

MANY early hospitals were for lepers and were called Lazar-houses. Leprosy, an Oriental disease, apparently as old as civilisation, prevailed extensively in Europe during the early Middle Ages. It would not be true to say that it was introduced into England as a new disease by the Crusaders, for it was known here before the Norman conquest. Pilgrimages to the Holy Land began in the fourth century and continued in an ever-increasing stream till 1064 (more than thirty years before the first Crusade), when we read of a host of seven thousand, accompanied by four bishops, most of which perished. Amongst those who were fortunate to return to their own homes, some, we may be sure, had become infected in the East with this pitiable disease and, its contagiousness not being at that time recognised, communicated it to others. The motive for providing retreats for lepers was not purely charitable, for the presence of these miserable outcasts in the streets and highways was regarded as repulsive, and many towns built lazar-houses for them. As just stated, the idea of contagion does not appear to have been at first realised, and other sick and destitute persons were admitted along with them. On the other hand, pity was the supreme feeling with some, notably with Maud, the queen of Henry I., for not only did she establish in

8

1118 a home for forty lepers but personally attended
to them, washing and kissing their feet and saying that
in so doing she was washing the feet of the Eternal King.
Henry III., who, like Edward the Confessor and
Henry VI., was more a churchman than a man of affairs,
is reported to have kissed the feet of lepers.

Harbledown.—Not content with freely providing for
the aged and feeble, Lanfranc founded, contemporaneously with St. John's (see Chap. X.), a house for lepers
at Harbledown, near Canterbury. Miss Clay gives a
drawing by Nelson, dated 1766, showing the ancient
church surrounded, at that time, by later wooden
buildings for the pensioners.[1] The lepers were not
allowed to wander about the town, but were permitted
to go beyond the precincts on specific business. Both
men and women wore russet-coloured garments, the
men having " scapulars or the ordinary working dress
of a monk " and hoods, the women thick veils. Both
wore ox-hide boots reaching half way up the leg.

At several lazar-houses, including Harbledown, there
were wells (springs), as at Burton Lazars, Peterborough,
Newark and Nantwich, which were credited with healing
powers. The holy well at Harbledown was called
" Black Prince's Well," and on the keystone of the
arch over it were carved the Prince's three feathers
and the words *Ich Dien*. After leprosy had become
less rife in England, an ecclesiastic dignitary refounded
Harbledown and, by his statutes, lodging, fuel and a
certain annual stipend were provided for thirty poor
honest men and thirty poor honest women. The house
was partly rebuilt at a later date, but a considerable

---

[1] Rotha Mary Clay, *op. cit.*

part of the Norman building remains with mural paintings. The floor of the church slopes downwards from east to west, probably for irrigation after the lepers had attended mass. The old seats and bench-ends are retained.

Erasmus, in his *Perigrinatio Religionis*, written about 1510, thus describes his visit to Harbledown with Colet, Dean of London :—

" On the left side of the road is an almshouse of some old men, one of whom runs out, as soon as they perceive a horseman approaching, and after sprinkling him with holy water, offers him the upper leather of a shoe bound with brass in which a piece of glass is set like a gem. This is kissed and money given to him. . . . The learned Dr. Colet, Dean of St. Paul's, rode on my left, nearer to the almshouse, and so he was sprinkled with the water ; to this he submitted but when the shoe was held out for him to kiss it, he asked what it meant and on being told it was the shoe of St. Thomas à Becket, he was sore provoked. . . . I took compassion on the old man and gave him some money by way of consolation."

This little picture of the two friends and equals in age throws an interesting " sidelight " on the thoughts and temper of each. Both deplorers of ignorance and despisers of superstition springing from it, the Dean manifests his disgust, while the greater man of letters and the humorist acts upon his instinct of sympathy. Noticing the shock to his beliefs and the pain of the old man, he drops a coin into his money-box : perhaps the same old box figured by Miss Clay and kept at Harbledown. This House of Pity still exists under the patronage of the Archbishops of Canterbury.

Queen Maud's Hospital.—On *Plate* XII. in Miss Clay's book, are reproduced a map, plan and sketch of date about 1566 and now in the British Museum. It shows how, even 400 years later, Queen Maud's Hospital was truly " in the fields " at Holborn. Here we see, within enclosing walls, several acres of land and fields and intersecting streets without. The church and infirmary stand apart, and there are an orchard, gardens, a pool and what may have been the master's house at that time. There is a round belfry-tower to the church, and the plan shows that it was divided into two parts by an east to west screen, one the parish church, the other the infirmary chapel.

This hospital was dedicated to St. Giles, the patron saint of lepers, himself reputed lame. He appears to have been a pre-Benedictine hermit living in a desert near Arles in Provence. In the twelfth century, St. Giles' shrine was a celebrated object of pilgrimage, while in England about one hundred and fifty churches and some twenty-five hospitals were dedicated to this saint, one of the former being at Cripplegate in London, while the ancient Cathedral of St. Giles in Edinburgh used to boast of possessing one of his bones. The legend of the wounded hart which, it was said, fled to him and supplied him with her milk, is perpetuated in the seals of the hospitals at Norwich, Wilton (a lazar-house) and Kepier, co. Durham.[1]

Burton Lazars, Leicestershire, was founded in 1146 by Roger de Mowbray, a Crusader, an adherent of King

[1] See description of the Seal of St. Giles, Norwich, Chap. IX.

Stephen and taken prisoner with him at the battle of Lincoln in 1141, and was dedicated to the Virgin Mary and St. Lazarus. This saint was identified with Lazarus, the brother of Martha and Mary of Bethany, and his association with lepers was derived, through some apparent confusion of the Gospel narratives, from the parable of Dives and Lazarus. It is remarkable that the seal of the post-Reformation hospital founded by Archbishop Whitgift at Croydon in 1596 depicts the " history " of Dives and Lazarus.[1] John Leland (c. 1506–52) speaks of Burton Lazars as " a very fine hospital and collegiate church." Queen Maud's hospital and others became affiliated to it.

Sherburn Hospital, co. Durham, was founded about 1181 by Bishop Puiset for sixty-five lepers in five " convents " of thirteen each.[2] The number thirteen, sometimes pretended at the present day to be " unlucky," was evidently not so regarded by the mediævals, for, as commemorating the Last Supper of their Lord, still with the purest in heart a cherished master, it was a practice, lasting through centuries, to specify that number. Miss Clay gives an illustration from Hutchinson's *Durham*, 1787, which shows the more important buildings of Sherburn on two sides of a quadrangle. It had a fair-sized detached church, *still in use*, as well as two chapels, one of which communicated with the quarters of the sick and infirm. In addition to the church, an ancient gateway remains and some of the work of the late Norman builders. Sherburn suffered much from the battle of Neville's Cross in 1346, when David II. of Scotland seized the opportunity of Edward III.'s

[1] See Fig. 23, p. 110.
[2] See detailed description of this hospital in Miss Clay's book.

absence with his army in France to invade the
Palatinate of Durham and, suffering signal defeat, was
taken prisoner. Leprosy having greatly decreased
by 1434, two places only were reserved for lepers at
Sherburn, *if they could be found*, the hospital assuming
more general functions. Unfortunately, Sherburn
suffered much from abuses, as was the case with many
another hospital, so that the number became reduced
to thirteen. Still, it somehow survived the Dissolution
and continues to be an almshouse with increasing
revenues. There were five other lazar-houses in London
besides Queen Maud's, outside the city walls, namely,
one of very early date, called St. James', for leprous
maidens, where are now the Palace and Park of that
name; at Stratford le Bow; at Knightsbridge;
between Shoreditch and Newington; and in Kent Street,
Southwark. This last is mentioned in the time of
Edward II., seems to have been of royal foundation
and was for a long time under the care of St. Bartholomew's Hospital. An illustration in Wilkinson's *Londinia Illustrata* shows its chapel used as a school in 1820.
Leprosy only died out gradually in England and
several lazar-houses were set up in the fourteenth
century.

CHAPTER III

YORKSHIRE

The First Hospital.—More than three hundred years after the advent of Augustine and his monks, that is, in 937, we find Athelstane, favourite grandson of Alfred the Great, returning from his victory in Dumfries over a confederacy of Scotch, Welsh and Scandinavians. He thus becomes " Rex totius Britanniæ " and assumes for the first time in English history the Greek title of " Basileus."[1] There being many needy pilgrims and travellers in the busy thoroughfare of YORK, besides other helpless persons, King Athelstane grants a site and considerable endowments to the canons of the Minster for founding a hospital to be dedicated to St. Peter. These funds were derived, *inter alia*, from a gift made to him by his northern subjects of *thraves*, henceforth called " Peter-corn," in recognition of his freeing their country of wolves. These thraves consisted of a proportion of the sheaves produced from every plough in Yorkshire, Cumberland, Westmorland and Lancashire.

Later, in 1155, we read of King Stephen refounding the hospital and rededicating it to St. Leonard after a great and destructive fire. This became a vast estab-

---

[1] *Encyc. Brit.*, " Æthelstane."

14

lishment maintaining, in 1370, two hundred and twenty-four sick and otherwise infirm inmates, besides orphans, and educating choir-boys in grammar and music. St. Leonard's had three chapels, and the ruins figured by Miss Clay[1] show a splendid ambulatory with octagonal pillars and pointed arches in the vaulting as well as remains of a large thirteenth-century apse to a chapel. Benefactions were conferred from time to time, Henry III. granting freedom to take timber from his Yorkshire forests, herbage and pasture and " anything useful for their use, as they had in the time of Henry II." So extensive and scattered were the estates of the hospital that a special clerk was required in their administration. According to Miss Clay, the constitution was more secular than ecclesiastic, and a layman might be the Warden. Notwithstanding the patronship of the canons of York Minster, supervision being probably but imperfectly maintained, many abuses crept in, which, with the woes of war and of pestilence, reduced the revenues and usefulness of the hospital, so that by 1462 the inmates numbered a hundred less than in 1370. At the Dissolution of the monasteries, Cromwell's commissioners reported that they had made certain " alterations," which practically amounted to annihilation. At the present day, a mere fragment of the foundation of a thousand years ago is represented by " cremitt money " (from *eremite*, a lonely man) distributed amongst thirty-one poor persons.

Besides the great hospital of St. Peter or St. Leonard there were thirteen others, as recorded in Dugdale's

[1] *Op. cit.*

Monasticon. The following is therein quoted from Bishop Tanner, an earlier writer. " There was in or near this city [York] an hospital for leprous persons as ancient as the time of Maud the Empress, who was a benefactor to it, and it is thought to be the same which was afterwards known by the name of St. Nicholas without Walmgate Barr, which was of royal foundation. It consisted of a Warden and several brothers and sisters." The last Warden was John Shirwode of the time of Edward IV. Here are the scanty records of the remaining twelve.

1. St. Anthony, founded about 100 years before Leland's time (*c.* 1506–52).
2. St. Mary the Greater, Bootham, 1314, by Robert Pykering, Dean of York, on the site of White Friars, which later became a hospital and, at the Dissolution, a school for the Dean and Chapter's scholars.
3. St. Mary the Less, Bootham, 1481, for two chaplains, etc.
4. At Fishergate, mentioned in 1399.
5. St. Giles, 1274.
6. Laithorpegate, founded by the Bigots. " Sir Francis Bigot let both the hospital and his house all to ruin "—Leland.
7 and 8. Two Maisons Dieu, one mentioned in the registers of Fountains Abbey.
9. Marygate Hospital.
10. Micklegate Hospital, begun but never finished.
11. St. Thomas the Martyr. This was still surviving in 1830 and, like one of the Maisons Dieu,

appears in the register of Fountains Abbey, to wit, in 1391. According to *Monasticon*, it was outside " Mickly Bar," in a suburb of York, but its founder is unknown.

12. In 1372, John de Ronclif, clerk, founded a hospital in Fossgate under letters patent of Edward III. for a master, thirteen poor infirm people, and two poor clergy to teach school. At Ronclif's death, however, there were not sufficient funds to carry out his intentions in full. We next hear of a company of York merchants endowing the hospital in the time of Henry VI. and of its being *still kept up* (1830) by the " Society of Merchant Adventurers " for ten poor widows.[1]

Pontefract, in the West Riding, has a rather curious history. If it was not actually a Roman settlement, remains of a Roman camp exist in the neighbourhood. The family of the De Lacys was long predominant. Ilbert de Lacy built a castle at Kirkby, said to be on the site of the fortified mound or "burgh" of Ailric, an Anglian thane. The ruins of the castle are on a rocky height, where were eight round towers and precincts covering more than eight acres, besides underground chambers cut in the native rock. At the date of Domesday Survey, Kirkby was subordinate to the Manor of Tateshall, but later the former became the borough of Pontefract, while the latter (now Tanshelf) remains a suburb. Before the Conquest, Robert de Lacy founded the hospital of St. Nicholas, which at the Dissolution

[1] *Monasticon.*

had a chaplain and thirteen poor people. It was " in being " as late, at least, as the seventeenth century. Sir Robert Knolles, at that time a citizen of London and afterwards a noted warrior in France, and his wife founded in 1385 a college or chantry and an almshouse for a master, two chaplains, and thirteen poor men and women. The hospital was *not dissolved* and the patronage was placed by Elizabeth with the corporation " according to the ancient foundation."

Fountains, celebrated for the lovely ruins of its Abbey, a few miles from the city of Ripon, has certain historical connections with hospitals. One was for relief of the poor of the district and for travellers as early as the time of Richard I., while two others, already recorded at York, are mentioned in the registers of the abbey.

Ripon.—Tanner mentions the hospital of St. Mary on the river Skell, founded by Thurston, Archbishop of York, who died in 1139, for a chaplain and sisters and all lepers in " Richmondshire." At the Dissolution, there were a master, two or three chaplains, and some brethren. Tanner also mentions St. Ann's on the Skell, but says nothing more about it. In *Monasticon* the hospital of St. John the Baptist is stated to have been founded by an Archbishop of York *before* 4th of King John, and to be " still in being."

Doncaster.—We have the very scanty records in *Monasticon* of two hospitals in this town; one of St. James in the early years of Henry III. for sick persons and lepers which, *before* the Dissolution, had degenerated into a free chapel and chantry ; the other quoted as St. Nicholas' in the Plea Rolls of Henry III. There was, besides, a lazar-house to St. Mary Magdalene, Archbishop John Romayne granting indulgences to its contributors in 1286.

Jesus Hospital, Rothwell, was founded in 1591, and therefore post-Reformation, by Owen Ragdale, school-master, for twenty to thirty poor men, who had ten shillings weekly and clothing. A flattened arch leads into a small quadrangle, on the further side of which another rather less flattened arch gives access to a rear-building. This is figured as still existing by Sidney Heath in his *Old English Houses of Alms.*

The ancient town of Beverley, in the East Riding of Yorkshire, is world-famous for its beautiful Minster, founded in the seventh or eighth century by St. John of Beverley, the provost of which, later, was Thomas à Becket. We do not know much of the hospital of St. Giles, save that it is supposed to have been founded by one Wulse, some time after the Conquest, and that it survived till the Dissolution, when but five poor people remained in it.

Kingston-upon-Hull, *i.e.,* **Hull.**—John Kingeston founded a Maison Dieu in 1345. In the same town, Michael de la Pole, created first Earl of Suffolk in 1385, founded about the same time a hospital for thirteen poor men and thirteen poor women. This was rebuilt in the time of Charles II., and is *still " in being."*

Selby's, also in Kingston, was founded about 1376 for twelve poor men, probably by Richard de Revenser, Archdeacon of Lincoln and Robert de Selby, his brother-in-law.

Northallerton.—St. James' Hospital is usually ascribed to Hugh Pursar, Bishop of Durham, in the times of Henry II. and Richard I. It is said that chaplains were appointed to pray for the soul of Phillip, the successor of Hugh Pursar. At the Dissolution, there were a master, four brethren, two sisters and nine poor people, and it became part of the endowment of Christ Church, Oxford. A Maison Dieu was founded in 1476 by Richard de Moore, draper, for thirteen poor men and women, and *was still existing in* 1830, under the patronage of the Earl of Carlisle.

Scarborough.—Henry II. gave lands towards the founding of the hospital of St. Thomas the Martyr, which was finished by the burgesses, who were also reputed to have built another to St. Nicholas, in both of which were brethren and sisters in the times of Edwards I. and II. Neither Tanner nor the editors of *Monasticon*, who quote him, could collect any further information on the matter.

WESTMORLAND

Brough.—The only house of pity in this county which calls for our attention is in this place, on the pass into Yorkshire, where John Bragskill, early in the sixteenth century, established a hospital and chapel with two beds for travellers and other poor people, dedicating it to the Virgin and St. Gabriel. There were two chaplains, one to teach children grammar and singing, the other to celebrate divine services. At the Dissolution, a pension of £7 4s. 4d. out of its revenues was granted for the continuance of the grammar school.

NORTHUMBERLAND

Newcastle.—Two ancient hospitals were dedicated to the Virgin : one near Westgate, for a master and six brethren, was as old as the time of Henry III. : the other, founded, as it is believed, by Henry I., but refounded and enlarged by Asselock of Killinghow about the later years of Henry II. Both these hospitals were united under a charter of 1612, and were thenceforth for a master and sundry poor persons placed therein by the Corporation. There was yet another, dedicated to St. Mary Magdalene, dating back to the time of Henry I. This likewise was reorganised in 1612, when the chapel of St. Thomas on the bridge over the Tyne was annexed to it. In 1830 there were a master and three poor brethren under the Corporation. Newcastle has thus the credit of *retaining* its hospitals.

Bolton, a village in this county, had, in the thirteenth century, a lazar-house for a master, three chaplains, thirteen leprous men and other lay brothers. The exceptional appointment of Thomas Goldington, clerk and *surgeon to the King* in 1330, is recorded.

DURHAM

Kepier Hospital, in the county of Durham, already mentioned on p. 11, was founded in 1112 by the notorious Ranulf " Flambard " and dedicated to St. Giles. This singular man of strong personality was execrated in his day, and nicknamed Flambard by the contemporary barons for his skill as a mischief-maker. A

C

mete minister to the violent and unscrupulous Rufus, he enriched himself and raised funds for the King by " farming " ecclesiastical benefices.   On the other hand, he was distinguished for his vast building achievements, both lay and ecclesiastic.   Kepier was a foundation for thirteen brethren and lasted till the Dissolution.   Miss Clay speaks of considerable remains, and figures the groined and vaulted gate-house.

The Hospital of St. Edmund at Gateshead was founded by Bishop Farnham, who incorporated an earlier foundation with it, about 1247.   Miss Clay figures the chapel, which alone remains.   It has been restored, and is now used for Divine Service.   It has the unusual feature of seven lancets at the east end, decreasing from the central light, and trefoil-headed blank arcades, while on the west front is a deeply recessed doorway.[1]

LANCASHIRE

The Vast City of Manchester does not possess a single ancient hospital, in the sense we are considering, but it has in the great free school known far and wide as **Chetham's Hospital,** a real house of pity.   Originally a Roman fortress, occupying possibly a British strong-hold, the place became in the thirteenth century the baronial hall of the Groslets, and in the fourteenth of the de la Warres, a family connection.   In 1422, Thomas, brother of the eleventh baron, founded a College in connection with the parish church, now the

---

[1] This exceptional number of lancets is seen in Ockham Church, Surrey.

PLATE II.

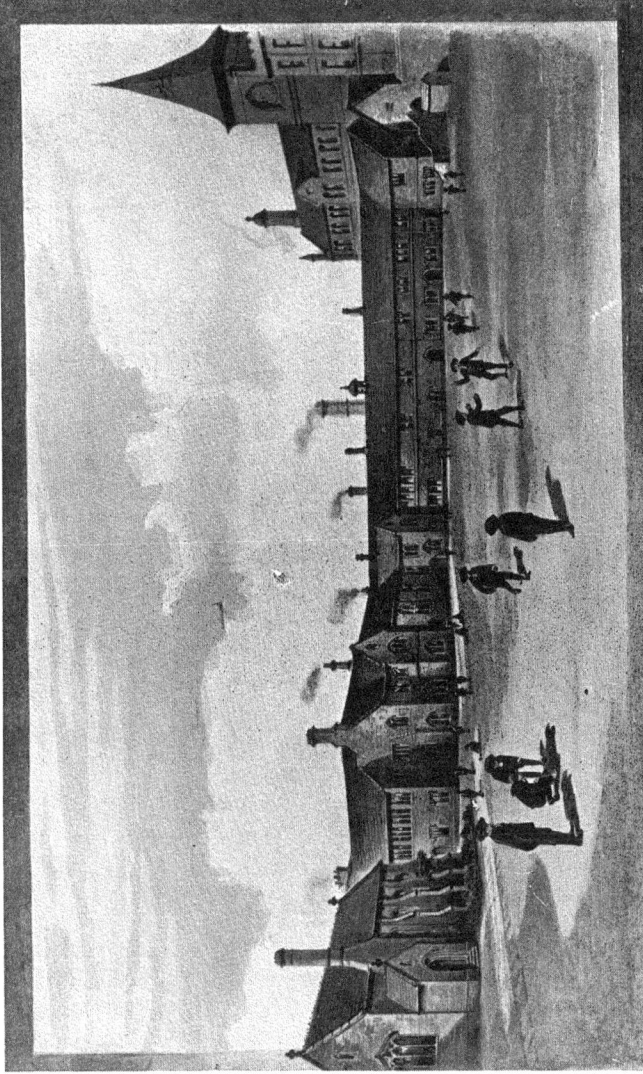

Fig. 2.—CHETHAM'S HOSPITAL.
By permission of Messrs Falkner, Manchester

[Face p. 22

Cathedral, and reconstructed his abode for the accommodation of its warden and fellows. Edward VI. dissolved the College, granting the hall to Edward Stanley, third Earl of Derby. Elizabeth restored the College and the fellows returned to their home as tenants of the Derby family. During the Civil War, Parliament sequestrated the place, dispossessing the ecclesiastics. Humphrey Chetham, a wealthy resident, bought the site and, in 1658, his trustees opened the school and a public library within it, which may be said to be the first free library in England. The ancient parts of this fine building furnish an interesting collection of mediæval and later constructions. The boys, now numbering 100, wear a costume resembling that of Christ Church *minus* the long skirt, except on state occasions, and a serviceable round flat cap.

CHAPTER IV

WARWICKSHIRE

Coventry.—Everybody has heard of Coventry, at least as a busy centre for the making of " cycles," " motors," etc., but, perchance, not every reader has realised its antiquity or heard of its ancient fame for trade in various stuffs.

The Warwickshire village of *Coventreu* owed its origin to the establishment of a Benedictine monastery in 1043 by Earl Leofric and his wife Godgyfu (the Lady Godiva of legend and Tennyson's sonnet). Too many of the old-world features have vanished before the hands of modern industrialism, yet venerable spires and towers still soar aloft, and many timber-framed houses remain from the ancient days.

Ford's Hospital.—Notably amongst these is the celebrated and much pictured Grey Friars' Hospital, not so called from any connection with the old Franciscan convent but because it stands in the street of that name. Lovely indeed in its unobtrusiveness is this little place of half-timbered homes, with their overhanging upper stories and carved wood-work, ranged around a narrow inner court.

Shortly before the Dissolution, namely in 1529, William Fourd, or Ford, founded this hospital for five

PLATE III.

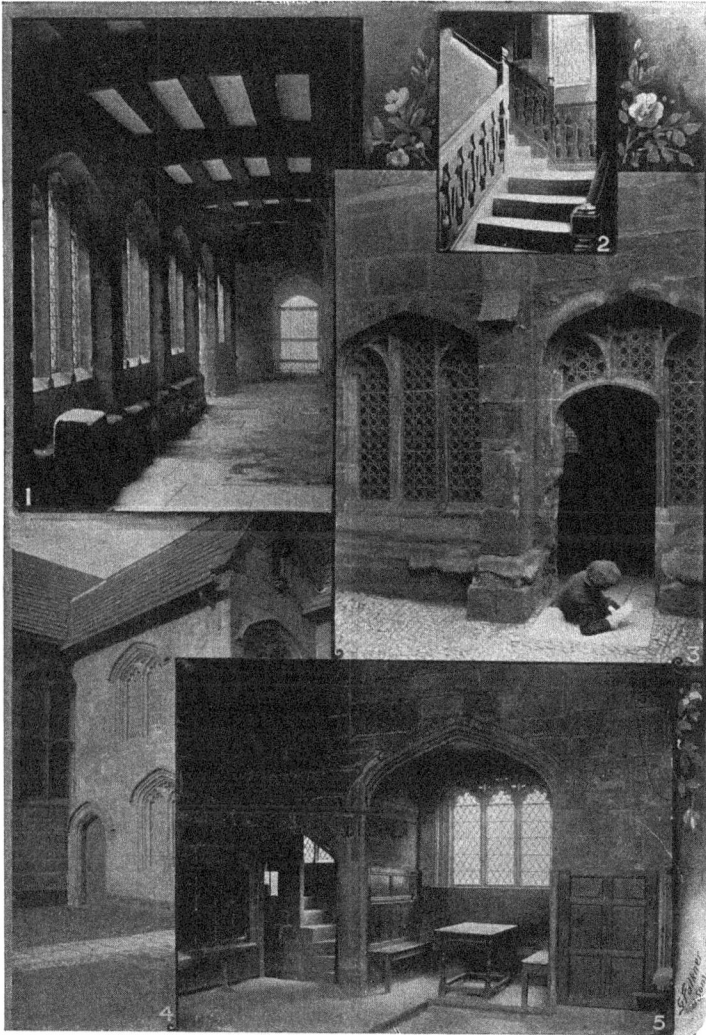

Fig. 3.—INTERIORS OF CHETHAM'S HOSPITAL
By permission of Messrs Falkner, Manchester

[Face p. 24

poor men and one woman, evidently placed there to tend the old men. William Pisford, Ford's executor, increased the number to *six men and their wives*, there being a later increase to seven married couples. If anyone should think to find in this a link with post-Reformation hospitals, he would be disappointed, for, as will be subsequently seen, the more *human* (if not more *humane*) feeling of Pisford is not apparent in *all* his sixteenth century successors. Ford, though on the eve of Henry's oscillating reformations, retained the belief in prayers for the departed, and provided for a priest to say mass twice a week for the souls of himself and his relations. This constituted his hospital a chantry, and was the excuse under the Act of Edward VI., though not carried into effect till the second year of James I., for its confiscation. Upon this, the city of Coventry purchased the forfeited estates from the Crown, and the hospital has ever since been maintained by the municipality. Later, the benefits became limited to women, and in 1908 there were 34 almswomen, 15 being residents, with a matron and sub-matron.[1]

With the death of Henry VIII. in 1547, we pass the border-line between the pre- and post-Reformation periods of hospital foundation. Yet we do not find any violent change in their constitution. It is true that founders did not declare, openly at any rate, their souls' health to be a motive ; no longer were the inmates to say a bidding prayer around their tomb ; the symbol of ancient faith manifest in dedication to patron saints disappeared; and, most notably and tangibly, the

---

[1] *Monasticon.* Sidney Heath, *op. cit. Victoria County History of Warwickshire. Encyc. Brit.,* " Coventry."

hospital chapel was no longer the pre-eminent architectural feature. Nevertheless, we find the traditional
number *thirteen*, as will be presently seen in Leicester's
hospital at Warwick, 25 years after Henry's death;
the hospital chapel, even if a subordinate part of the
fabric, surviving with strict rules of attendance there
and of marching in bede-gowns to the parish church;
while some ecclesiastic founders expected the pensioners
to be single persons. Structurally, too, the mediæval
custom of a college with buildings ranged round a
quadrangle and inner and outer gate-houses continued.

Bablake Hospital, founded by Thomas Bond, draper
and Mayor of Coventry in 1506, was for a priest, ten
poor men and one poor woman. It was granted by
Edward VI. to the Corporation and *still exists*, and
presents fine wood-carving.

The Hospital of St. John the Baptist was established
early in the reign of Henry II. with the consent and on
the soil of the Prior and Convent of Coventry, Edmund,
Archdeacon of Lichfield, bearing the principal cost.
It was for a master and several brethren and sisters,
and is said in its charter to have been founded as a
house of " perpetual pity " for the support of the poor
and infirm. It suffered dissolution, but a grammar
school took its place.

Warwick.—The predecessors of Elizabeth's favourite,
Robert Dudley, had long before established hospitals
in this town. One to St. John the Baptist was founded
by William, Earl of Warwick, in the time of Henry II.,
for strangers and pilgrims as well as for the poor and
infirm. Still earlier, in the reign of Stephen, Roger,
Earl of Warwick, built St. Nicholas' at the lower end

of Saltford Street for lepers. Leland says that in his time the buildings were "sore decayed."

Leicester Hospital was originally built for the Guilds of Holy Trinity and St. George in the fifteenth century. At the Dissolution, the property was acquired by the town and conveyed by deed of gift to Robert Dudley, Earl of Leicester, in 1571. He established the *present* hospital for a master and twelve men, preferably old soldiers, born in the counties of Warwick or Gloucester, or who had lived there for five years. Failing old soldiers, the pensioners were to be drawn from the poor of Kenilworth, Stratford-on-Avon, Wootton-under-edge, or Erlingham. The hospital was richly endowed by farms and tithes in the above-mentioned counties. By an Act of Parliament of 1813, the master received £400 per annum and the brethren £80 each.

The old buildings are very picturesque ; timbered houses with overhanging upper stories bearing the arms and badges of the Leicester and Warwick families ; a cloister by the side of the quadrangle; and the hall with fine chestnut roof. The church, in this a distinctive feature, stands a little apart, above the west gate of the ancient town wall, as the east gate is likewise surmounted, as was the case at Canterbury and Bristol, and is still at Winchester. A perpendicular screen separates the choir, within which the master and brethren have their stalls.

WORCESTERSHIRE

Worcester.—Two Anglo-Saxon bishops, St. Oswald and St. Wulfstan, are credited with the foundation of hospitals in this city. Leland says that St. Oswald's hospital was first for monks, then for lepers, afterwards a hospital for poor folk, with a master and fellows, and, finally, became a free chapel. It was demolished in time of Elizabeth, but was restored by Bishop Fell in the reign of Charles II. " in a sumptuous manner and recovered many of its possessions and *still maintains* twelve poor men." (*Monasticon*.)

HEREFORDSHIRE

The Cathedral City of Hereford had seven hospitals which are mentioned in *Monasticon*. The *Encyc. Brit.*, in the article " Hereford," however, mentions but two old hospitals as *existing*. Coningsby Hospital, founded by Sir T. Coningsby in 1614, has the distinction of its inmates wearing a " remarkable uniform of red, designed by the founder." St. Ethelbert's is a thirteenth century foundation.

DERBYSHIRE

Bentley.—Walter Blount, Lord Mountjoy, left by will, 1474, lands of £10 per annum to the then ancient hospital of St. Leonard, between Alkmanton and Bentley, for seventeen poor men not under the age of 55, old territorial servants being preferred, and provided for them pasture for seven cows, fuel from his manors, and a gown and hood every three years. These poor men were to pray for his soul and the soul of his family and ancestors, the souls of the Duke of Buckingham, Earl Rivers, Sir John Woodville, and the ancient lords of the hospital, and had to repeat, twice daily, the Psalter of the Virgin Mary. Lord Mountjoy also directed the building of a chapel at Alkmanton, where the master of the hospital was to celebrate mass once a year. *Monasticon* gives no account of the origin of this hospital. It disappeared after 1547, and *no vestiges*, save this record, remain.

LEICESTERSHIRE

Leicester.—In 1330, Henry, Earl of Leicester and Lancaster, and a grandson of Henry III., began to build his hospital of the Annunciation near his castle. Henry, Duke of Lancaster, augmented his father's work, giving it the distinctive name of " Newark College," and John of Gaunt further increased it. Its constitution was a Dean, 12 secular canons, 12 vicars, 3 clerks, 6 choristers, *one hundred* poor men, 10 nurses, etc. Leland, describing the College in his time, speaks of the large almshouse within the quadrangle, the "large and fair cloister," the " stately walls and gates," and the " exceeding fair " church. This last was demolished before 1590, but the hospital was suffered to *remain, as was also* Wiggeston's hospital (1513) in the same town, referred to later in connection with Sherborne, Dorset, and with East Hendred, Berks.

St. Ursula's was founded in the latter part of Henry VI.'s reign, or in that of Henry VII. *Monasticon* speaks of it as " *still under the patronage* of the Chancellor of the Duchy of Lancaster," but says nothing of its constitution.

Lutterworth, ever associated in gracious memory with England's pre-Reformer, John Wycliff, *retains* its ancient hospital of St. John the Baptist. Roise de Verdon and Nicholas, her son, built and endowed it in the time of King John for a master and brethren. In Queen Elizabeth's reign the mastership became vested in the hands of the Crown.

RUTLANDSHIRE

Oakham (of the horse-shoes) has a hospital founded by Wm. Dalby, merchant, in 1398, for 12 poor men with two chaplains, one to be warden, which is " *still in being.*"

In the same small county is Jesus Hospital. It had its origin in a country house of the bishops of Lincoln which, in 1602, was converted into a hospital by Thomas, Baron Burghley, for a Warden, 12 poor men and 2 poor women. The original great hall is intact and contains a flat ceiling, oriel window and large open fire-place, over which are the arms of Bishop Russell, who rebuilt the place towards the end of the sixteenth century. There is a cloister on the north with wooden supports to its roof.[1]

NORTHAMPTONSHIRE

Northampton.—St. John's is supposed to have been founded by William, Archdeacon of Peterborough,

---

[1] Sidney Heath *op. cit.*

about 1168, though the erection may have taken place after his death. It was for a master, two co-brothers, and eight poor men. Cubicles were arranged on either side of the hall, but the chapel at the north-east was only entered from the outside. It is now extinct, the funds having been dissipated through the peculations of masters in the seventeenth and eighteenth centuries.

Peterborough.—The cathedral city had once two hospitals. St. Leonard's for sick and leprous persons, was dependent upon the Abbey as early as Stephen's time. St. Thomas' is noteworthy as being one, if not the first, of the dedications to the Martyr. It was founded by Benedict, Abbot of Peterborough, who had been Prior of Canterbury and Chancellor to Beckett, about 1180, " to the honour of his old master, who now began to be accounted a saint and a martyr." (*Monasticon.*)

Higham Ferrers.—Henry Chicheley (1364–1443), Archbishop of Canterbury, established a bedehouse in this, his native town. Upon an older fourteenth century foundation, Chicheley instituted his bede-house in 1425, attaching to it a collegiate school. This high ecclesiastic, though he did not keep his hands from falling heavily upon the Lollards, must be credited with a genuine respect for learning. Besides Higham Ferrers, he founded St. Bernard's (since dissolved) and All Souls', Oxford. Croydon was one of the country manors of the See, and the noble western tower of the parish church is of Chicheley's building. He is the Archbishop of Shakespeare's *King Henry V.*, who is represented as encouraging the King's invasion of

France, though there appears to be no contemporary evidence of Chicheley's part in that scene.[1]

The hall at Higham Ferrers has an open roof springing from oaken corbels and a large original fireplace on its south side, while an arch divides it from the chapel at its eastern end. This is thus an example of the infirmary type, as we shall see elsewhere. The twelve bedesmen were directed by Chicheley's statutes to stand, each at his cubicle door, and join in evensong. The number of thirteen was completed by a woman who acted as matron with minutely defined duties. This house of pity *still exists*.

All Saints', Stamford, on the border of Northampton, but actually in Lincolnshire, was founded as a bedehouse in 1485 by William Browne, a rich merchant. Miss Clay figures it with its chapel under one roof. The dormitories of the bedesmen, on the ground-floor of the hall, communicate directly with the chapel, while the upper storey overlooks it from a gallery, the division being " a mere screen." The entire set of buildings are arranged around an inner court.

Banbury.—Tanner says that in the time of King John, a hospital was here founded and dedicated to St. John for a prior or master and several leprous brethren and sisters, the mastership being in the gift of the Bishop of Lincoln. The hospital was converted bodily into a school in 1501, and in 1541 Nicholas Cartwright, D.D., was presented to the mastership.[2] *Monasticon* states that the hospital stood at the foot of the bridge within the bounds of Warkworth, *i.e.*, on

---

[1] *Encyc. Brit.*, " Chicheley," by A. F. Leach.
[2] *Encyc. Brit.* makes this statement as to conversion, and says it was " a precedent frequently followed since."

the other side of the river Cherwell, and therefore in Northamptonshire.

STAFFORDSHIRE

The Cathedral City of Lichfield has a hospital " *still in being.*" St. John the Baptist's was originally a religious house. In the time of Henry VII., Bishop Smith refounded it for a master, two priests and ten poor men, the King himself being a great benefactor. At the time of the Dissolution there were thirteen poor persons, a bailiff, a schoolmaster and an usher.

NOTTINGHAMSHIRE

Nottingham.—John Plumtree of this town founded a hospital at Bridge-end, under licence of Richard II., for two chaplains, one to be master, and thirteen poor and aged widows, to the honour of the Annunciation. The founder himself reduced the number, but his descendants restored it to its original thirteen. *It is still " in being."*

BEDFORDSHIRE

Bedford, the county town of one of the smallest English shires, is always associated in our minds with "The Pilgrim's Progress," and John Bunyan, who dreamt his dream in Bedford Gaol. The river Ouse flows through this fertile county, and the "Great Escarpment" of the Chilterns, as they trend north-east, bound it from Hertford.

The Hospital of St. John the Baptist was founded in 1280 by Robert Parys for a master, two or more brethren-priests, and for the reception of decayed freemen of the town. Many years before the Reformation it ceased to be occupied according to the founder's direction. In 1830 co-brethren were appointed by the master, and received the *liberal* allowance of ninepence weekly without residence. The old hall is still standing.

St. Leonard's Hospital was established before 1302 by the townsmen, originally for three lepers, and was revived in 1889 and fully equipped as a modern hospital.

CHAPTER V

THE WEST SAXON KINGDOM

WE are not particularly concerned here with the first landing in Britain of that confederacy of invaders who called themselves, not Saxons, but Gewissas. Certain it is that they gradually made themselves masters of the whole south coast and far inland between the basins of the Warwickshire Avon and the Thames. We will place first in our group the great and sea-swept county of

DEVONSHIRE

Exeter.—As we would expect in a cathedral city, there were several houses of pity, to wit, three hospitals and three lazar-houses. God's House was founded in 1436 by Wynard, recorder of Exeter. A non-resident school was attached, in which children were taught the alphabet and the " great Psalter of Holy David." The chapel and the hospital *still exist*.

St. Katharine's, in Locks Lane, was founded in 1407 by the will of Sir Thomas Bonville, but the chapel only remains and is used by the Church Army.

William Prodem, a citizen of Exeter, founded the Hospital of St. Alexius in 1170, behind the Priory of St. Nicholas, for poor persons. It was incorporated with St. John's Hospital soon after 1230, but an impression of its seal, reading in English : " The seal of the hospital behind St. Nicholas," is retained in the archives of the city.

St. John the Baptist's was established about 1230 by the brothers, Gilbert and John Long, near the east gate of the city, for poor men and women and, soon after St. Alexius was incorporated with it, John entered and became the superior. The patronage was first in the hands of the citizens, but in 1244 they exchanged it with the Bishop of Exeter for that of St. Giles' lazar-house, at the south gate. Thenceforth, till its extinction at the Dissolution, the Bishops of Exeter, in the main, gave good care to the hospital and bestowed benefactions upon it. Bishop Grandison was pre-eminent amongst these. Finding the place in a deplorable condition, reduced to one priest and a few invalids, he raised the clergy to five and the pensioners to twelve, rebuilt the church and attached a free resident school. The last prior, Richard Harrys, subscribed to the King's supremacy with three of his brethren in 1534, and surrendered the hospital to Henry on February, 1539. Tanner says that the site, with an " ankeresse-house " in the churchyard, was granted by the King to Thomas Carew, but that the hospital was afterwards restored, endowed with several benefactions, and *continued* under the management of the city. Grandison's school was restored by the Crossing family in 1669.

Tavistock.—Tanner states that by patents of Edward III. and the register of Bishop Lacy, a hospital appears to have been founded for lepers and dedicated to St. Mary Magdalene.

Leland, writing in the time of Henry VIII., speaks of a hospital then standing in the heart of the town, and supposed to have been founded by one Ake. He goes on to narrate that " ther is an Hospitale of the foundation of two Marchant men, Akebarrow and Hodgekin Overstal, standyng hard without the North Bargate." This was the decayed hospital of St. Nicholas, mentioned in 1286 and in the times of Edward III. and Richard II.

WILTSHIRE

Devizes.—Tanner mentions two hospitals, " now under the government of the Mayor and Corporation, but perhaps formerly in the patronage of the King." One of these was founded for lepers before 1207.

Salisbury.—Harnham Hospital *still exists*. Dedicated to St. Nicholas, it is said to have been founded by Herbert or Richard Poore, Bishop of Salisbury, about 1220, close to the bridge of that name, for eight poor men and four poor women. Restored by James I. in 1610, it has a clerical master, nominated by the Bishop and still maintains twelve inmates, one being nominated by the Dean and Chapter, the rest by the master. Holy Trinity, attributed to John Chandler, about 1394, was for twelve poor men and *remains* under the Corporation.

Wilton, the county town, has the *credit of still preserving* two ancient hospitals. The founding of St. Julian's is by tradition ascribed to Henry I.'s second wife, Alicia, who is buried there. It was early in the patronage of the Corporation, and was not dissolved, and though rebuilt by them in 1624, was in great decay in Tanner's time. There are a master, who is a clergyman, and four poor people.

D

St. John's was founded in 1217, or earlier, by one Hubert, who cannot be certainly identified with the Bishop of Sarum elevated in 1187 to the Archbishopric of Canterbury. It *still stands* near the gate of the town, and provides a home for two poor men and two poor women under a clerical master.

GLOUCESTERSHIRE

Cirencester.—*Monasticon* mentions *two small hospitals as existing* in 1830, namely, St. John the Evangelist's, from Henry I.'s time, for three poor men and three poor women, and that of St. Laurence, of Edward III.'s time, with two poor women and a master.

Gloucester was not originally a cathedral city, there being so long ago as 681 an Abbey of St. Peter, the foundations of the present church being laid by Abbot Serlo in the late years of the eleventh century or the early of the twelfth. In 1541 it was constituted a cathedral by Henry VIII. Gloucester, like Wilton, *has retained* its old houses of pity. St. Margaret's was a lazar-house before 1320, and in 1830 maintained nine poor people, while St. Mary Magdalene's had nineteen. St. Bartholomew's, near the city, had its origin in a house built for the men employed in some constructive work, and continued for poor sick workmen till the time of Henry III. There were, in 1830, twenty-four men pensioners and thirty women, with a master, minister, physician, surgeon, and an income of £500 per annum.

Bristol.—This great city and ancient port has had several hospitals, some of which have perished or been transformed.

St. Bartholomew's, a short distance from Grey Friars', outside Frome Gate, was, after the Dissolution, conveyed to the Corporation for a grammar school, which still exists. In Lyon's Hospital, a few poor people *still reside* under the direction of St. James' parish, while in the hospital founded by John Foster *there are* eight men and five women under the Corporation. *Monasticon* has words practically identical with the following : Hard within Lawford's gate was a hospital believed to have been founded in fourth Henry V., by John Barnstaple, merchant of Bristol, for six poor men, six poor women and a priest ; but Tanner says there was certainly an earlier foundation before Henry's time, though probably not fully settled. Hence we may infer that the hospital was here in the fourteenth century. *It was not dissolved,* and was granted by Elizabeth to the Corporation, who greatly improved the revenues.

SOMERSET

Bath.—The hospital of St. John the Baptist is *still existing.* It was founded by Reginald, Bishop of Bath, about 1180, for succour of the poor who resorted to the Cross and the Hot Baths. The masters appear to have been presented by the Priors of Bath Abbey. Queen Elizabeth gave the advowson to the Corporation of that city.

The little hospital of St. Mary Magdalene FOR LUNATICS is said to have been built by John Canton, who was Prior of Bath from 1489 to 1499. It survived the Dissolution, " but gradually became a sinecure, its endowments being diverted from their original purpose " (*Victoria County History*, from Bath Municipal Records).

Glastonbury.—Although there is now no old hospital in this place, unless the Women's Almshouse mentioned by Miss Clay is such, the peculiar interests gathered around this ancient shrine call for a passing notice of a home for poor and infirm people, under the care of the Almoner of Glastonbury, and dedicated, like many another, to St. John the Baptist. Michael, Abbot of that house, rebuilt it in 1246 near the park, increased the allowances for the poor, and provided a chaplain.

Bridgwater.—Formerly, there were two ancient hospitals, neither of which now exists. Leland says of one, St. John the Baptist's, that the house which was standing in his day had, previously, secular priests who bore a cross on the breast, and that a hospital adjoined. Tanner says that it was founded before 1214, and that, besides the poor, pilgrims were entertained. Needless to say, it was dissolved. The Seal attached to the acknowledgment of Henry's supremacy is in the Chapter House of Westminster, and is thus described in the British Museum Catalogue of Seals : " On a bridge of 4 arches over a river, the Virgin and Child between St. John the Baptist holding an Agnus Dei and (?) St. Paul with a book in his left hand and a sword in his right, all full length under a canopy." Only a small portion of ruins were to be seen in 1830.

CHAPTER VI

West Saxon Kingdom—*continued*

DORSETSHIRE

Sherborne has a hospital, which was established in 1437, upon an earlier foundation, by Robert, Bishop of Salisbury, Sir Humphrey Stafford, and others for twenty brethren, twenty poor and impotent men, four women and a chaplain. A master, moreover, was to be chosen from among the brethren and the whole governed by statutes enacted by the community. This scheme, which looks like an early experiment in democracy, does not seem to have been a success, for we read of the property being " filched away piece-meal." All the same, the hospital *remains to this day* as an actual building of the fifteenth century, with hall, chapel, and other parts, and is figured in Parker's *Ancient Domestic Architecture.* It presents an example of the common arrangement in domestic chapels, as is also seen in All Saints', Stamford; Wiggeston's Hospital, Leicester; and East Hendred, mentioned on pp. 29 and 64. At Sherborne, both stories communicated with the chapel, which was separated by a screen, the men sitting on the ground-floor, the women on the upper floor. This hospital was dedicated to St. John the Baptist and St. John the Evangelist.

Wimborne is a little old-fashioned country town in the heart of " Hardy Land," and was at one time the residence of that great man of letters. It is situated on the beautiful river Allen, close to its confluence with the Stour, its commanding feature being the grand Norman Minster. This is of very early foundation, for it is stated in the Anglo-Saxon Chronicle that Cuthburh (later canonised as St. Cuthberga, to whom a church on the site was afterwards dedicated) did found at Wimburn an Abbey in 718, of which she was the first superior. The Abbey was probably destroyed by the Danes, and Edward the Confessor founded thereafter a College of secular canons.

About half a mile from the Minster, by the road-side and on a little hill, is a cluster of thatched and other cottages and a small church, in a garden. This is St. Margaret's Hospital, founded in or about 1241, as it appears according to Tanner, by the lords of the manor of Kingston Lacy, in whom it is vested. There are nine tenements, three for single men, three for single women, and three for married couples. By the chapel door is a holy-water stoop, too high up now to be easily examined, but said by Mr. Sidney Heath to be worn down at its edge by countless fingers. Inside, remains of mural paintings are to be seen on the walls.

HAMPSHIRE

Basingstoke.—Walter de Merton, so called from his close association with the Priory at Merton in Surrey, was the founder of the College at Oxford which bears his name. He also established a hospital at Basing-stoke, where he was born or, at least, his parents had

PLATE IV.

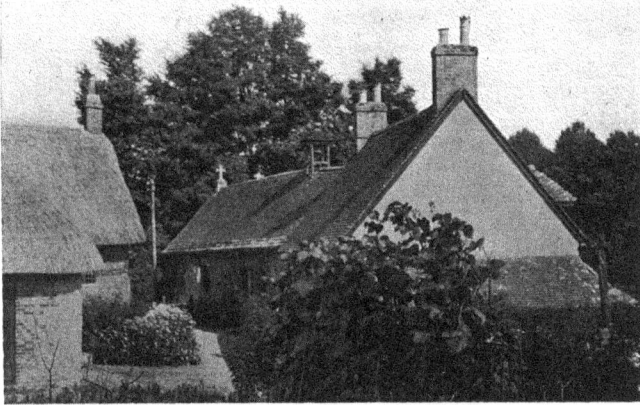

Fig. 4.—ST. MARGARET'S, WIMBORNE

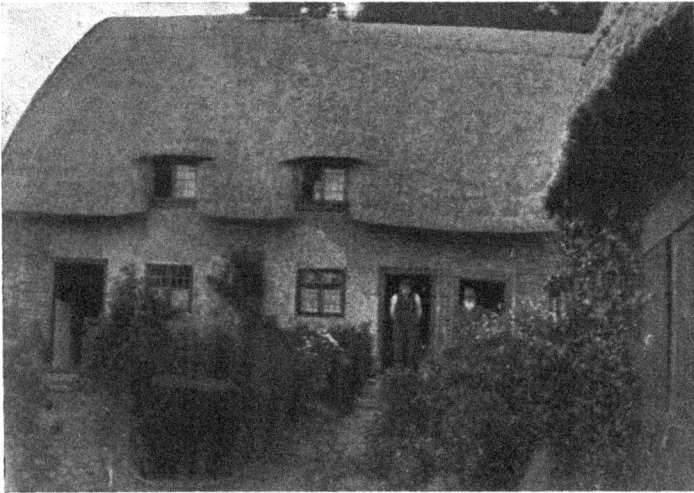

Fig. 5.—ST. MARGARET'S, WIMBORNE

[*Face p. 42*

resided, chiefly for the benefit of poor clergy. It was appointed that the incurably sick scholars at Merton College should be placed there, and the mastership of both places was combined. The hospital was rebuilt in 1778, and *still exists*.

Southampton.—Two brothers, Gervasus and Protusius, converted their own dwelling into a God's-house in the time of Henry III., dedicating it to St. Julian. It *still exists* and is figured by Miss Clay.

Portsmouth.—Peter de Rupibus, Bishop of Winchester, established, in the time of King John, a God's-house and dedicated it to St. John the Baptist and St. Nicholas. It is now the Garrison Church.

Winchester.—The author is indebted to Mr. Kenneth A. Ryde, M.C., Chief of Reference Department at Croydon Free Library, for the following account of England's first Capital.

The grand old city, with its cathedral and other ancient buildings, lies snugly in the lap of the chalk downs of mid-Hampshire, and is watered by the pretty river Itchin which meanders along its way to Southampton Water. Its legendary, historical, ecclesiastical and literary associations are manifold. The very early history of Winchester is lost in the remote past, but the surrounding hills preserve the vestiges of vanished peoples in the shape of earthworks and barrows. This early British place was known as Caer Gwent. The Romans, who called it Venta Belgarum, from the tribe of Belgae, which they found in that part of Britain, have left ample evidence of their occupation. No less than six Roman roads radiate from the city, showing that it must have been a place of great importance, while many relics have been discovered, including coins, pavements and the foundations of houses.

After the departure of the Romans, the Gewissas or West Saxon confederates, under Cerdic, conquered Hampshire early in the sixth century, making the Roman Venta the capital of the Wessex Kingdom. It is said that from this first King of Wessex are descended nearly all our English kings. Thereafter, Venta became Vintan-ceaster, which survives in " Winton," the ecclesiastical style of the Bishop, and here, in 827, Egbert was crowned King of all England, making the place we now know as Winchester the capital of the whole country.[1]

The Cathedral occupies the site of two former Christian churches. One erected by King Kynegils of the West Saxons, completed by his son Kenwalh in 648, and dedicated to SS. Peter and Paul, and the other by King Ethelwold in 980 and dedicated to St. Swithin. Ethelwold died in 984 and was buried in the church he had built, which was known as the Old Minster. The plan and foundations of the present cathedral are the

[1] *Caer* is without question Celtic, meaning a fortress, and has, maybe, a root common to it and the Latin *castrum*, from whence comes our word *castle*. As to *Gwent*, the opinions of etymologists are divided. Putting on one side the ideas of such old writers as Leland and Camden, who would have it to mean *white*, as such places on the chalk would suggest, one finds Johnston, in his *Place-names of England and Wales*, rendering *venta* and *gwent* as an open place or clearing, but quoting M'Clure as saying that *Venta* means a market, and is not Celtic, but late Latin, from *vendere*, *venditum*, whence our word vendor. The Welsh-English Dictionary also gives *gwent* as " a fair or open region, now confined to nearly all Monmouthshire, but anciently including parts of Gloucester and Hereford, being a district where Caer Went or Venta Silurum of the Romans was the capital." The Romans named several places Venta, adding a tribal qualification, such as Venta Belgarum, V. Icenorum (Caister near Norwich), Venta Silurum. If we accept Johnston's and the Welsh Dictionary's rendering, we must take the entire word *Caer Gwent* as Celtic, and suppose that the Romans, finding certain places called *gwent* by the British, Latinised them into Venta. On the other hand, if we follow M'Clure, we have to assume that the natives, as they became Romanised, copied *venta* as gwent just as the Anglo-Saxons later adopted *caer* or *castrum* as ceaster —J. M. H.

work of Bishop Walkelyn, a cousin of the Conqueror. It was begun in 1079, and took fourteen years to build.[1] It far exceeded the dimensions of the Old Minster, which had been much damaged by the Danes.

About the year 1200, Bishop Godfrey de Lucy added the eastern end of the cathedral and, in the fourteenth century, Bishop Edyngdon began, and Bishop William of Wykeham completed, the transformation of the Norman nave into the finest perpendicular nave in Britain. Winchester is the longest cathedral in England (556 ft.), and the second longest in Europe. Its beauty is to be found in its interior, not in its exterior. As one enters by the west door, the vista is very striking, and has been considered unequalled. At the west end of the north aisle is the oldest piece of iron grille-work in England, dating from the eleventh century. The font is of black Tournai marble of about 1180, the sculptures on its south and west sides representing scenes from the life of St. Nicholas of Myra. The beautiful west window was originally glazed about 1385, but it was much damaged in Cromwell's time, and only fragments of the early glass remain. The splendid reredos is of late fifteenth or early sixteenth century, and is from its style attributable to Bishop Fox, who also erected that in Southwark Cathedral. Winchester is famous for the number and the beauty of its shrines, which are gems of architectural design. Amongst these chantry chapels are those of Bishops Edyngdon (1366), William of Wykeham (1404), Cardinal Beaufort (1447), Wayneflete (1486) and Fox (1528). The lovely shrine of St. Swithin was destroyed in 1539. Besides

[1] Early Norman work exists in the transepts.—J. M. H.

these are the last resting-places of many great personages, in which respect only Westminster and St. Paul's
can compare.

Besides the Old Minster, whose site is occupied by
the Cathedral, a New Minster was built close by at
the request of Alfred by his son, Edward the Elder, in
903. In 1110 it was removed to Hyde, the monks
taking with them the remains of Alfred. The Abbey of
Hyde, as it was called, thrived till the Dissolution, but
all that remains of it at the present day is a fourteenth
century gateway.

After all, the greatest name connected with Winchester is that of King Alfred, the " Father of English
prose." He began to reign in 871, and in his later years
made the city his home. He held his court here, and
gathered around him scholars from near and far for
the advancement of learning and to educate his people.
From Winchester the Witan issued its decrees, and here
Alfred studied, laboured, and began the Anglo-Saxon
Chronicle, the treasured record of contemporary history.
He died in 901, and his remains have been three times
interred, first in the Old Minster, next in the New
Minster, and, lastly, in Hyde Abbey. Yet where his
bones lie " no man knoweth," for at the destruction
of the Abbey his tomb was lost. In 1901, Alfred's
millennium was celebrated, and an eloquent bronze
statue of him, close to the modern Guildhall, was
unveiled.[1]

The ruins of Wolvesey Castle are near the cathedral ;
in Saxon times a palace stood here, where Alfred the

---

[1] When we come to Berkshire, we shall see that another statue, in stone and
in my view, better characteristic of the man, had already been erected at
Wantage, his birth-place, in 1877.—J. M. H.

Great lived. After the destruction of this palace, Bishop Henry de Blois built a castle on the spot, in 1138, and here he resisted the forces of Queen Matilda, and here many historical events took place. It was for several centuries the seat of the Bishops of Winchester, but was destroyed in 1646, during the Civil War. Later, in 1665, Bishop Morley and his successors built a residence there, the main part being demolished by Bishop North in the eighteenth century, leaving the chapel, which is now the Diocesan Church House.

Winchester Castle, near the West Gate, is a Norman foundation, rebuilt by Henry III., and also destroyed by Cromwell in 1646, except the Castle Hall, now the County Hall. Many events of historical importance occurred here, including the first Parliaments of England, 1265, state-trials, etc. In the Hall is preserved a round table, said to be over 700 years old, and, by tradition, the actual table of Arthur and his knights. William of Wykeham is so well known as a great man that no more need be said of him, save that he founded Winchester College in 1384, the oldest in England, still a famous school, and entitling him to be called the " Father of the English public school system."

The West Gate is one of the two remaining of the five city gates, and dates from the fourteenth century. The other is King's Gate, and is surmounted by the little church of St. Swithin, reminding us of similarly placed churches at Warwick, Bristol and Canterbury (see p. 27). The curfew bell is still rung nightly, and the " oldest house " was a rectory-house, double-gabled, and built in the early sixteenth century.

The Hospital of the Holy Cross.—Winchester is a

city teeming with memories and old survivals of a long
distant past. Walking down the High Street, passing
the statue of Alfred the Great, who holds aloft his
sword, like a cross, we presently traverse the bridge
over the clear and swift river Itchin. A few steps
further and we reach the " oldest house " above
mentioned, and thence, following the walls of the
ancient castle and passing Bishop Wykeham's College,
we rejoin the banks of the brimming river. Then, all
at once, the noble pile of the Hospital of the Holy Cross
comes into view. This may fitly be called the
Premier Hospital of England, for, though not the oldest
extant, it has preserved nigh intact the form given it
by its founders.

Henry de Blois, Bishop of Winchester, founded St.
Cross about 1136 for thirteen poor men. He, the son
of Stephen, Count de Blois in France, and brother of
Stephen, King of England, was an advocate of the
highest claims of the Church and, while he held the
office of the Pope's legate, the greatest ecclesiastic in
England. It was not altogether unusual for a churchman of the Middle Ages to assume the character of a
warrior, and Henry was one of these. His defence of
Winchester against the Empress Matilda, as already
mentioned by Mr. Ryde, and on the side of his brother
Stephen, was the turning point in the civil war of that
time. Besides his foundation of St. Cross, he built
several castles, of which that at Farnham, Surrey, is
still the seat of the Bishops of Winchester.

De Blois' frankly expressed motives in founding his
hospital may be taken as typical of the mediæval mind
in these matters. Thus : " Which I, for the health of

my soul and the souls of my predecessors and of the kings of England have founded . . . that the poor in Christ may there humbly and devoutly serve God."[1] De Blois also provided that a hundred poor men of good character should have a substantial meal every day, and the ancient custom of a dole of bread and beer to all comers is continued, in a limited extent, to the present time.

St. Cross has survived its chequered fortunes. The intention of de Blois was that the Knights Hospitallers should be the controllers and administrators of his hospital, and in his charter of 1151 he handed over its charge to Raymond du Puy, Grand Master at Jerusalem, and his successors " for ever." The immediate occasion for this act may have been the existence of a preceptory of the Knights at Baddesley, near Lymington, in the same county. The Bishop seems to have appointed the first Master, Robert de Limosia, though he evidently considered the office quite subordinate to the control of the Hospitallers. This, however, led later to a long-drawn dispute between the Bishop of Winchester and the Knights, which only ended in 1204. Since then, the Bishops have always appointed the master, and the connection with the Knights eventually ceased. Looking back, de Blois' ideal seems natural. He, an ardent churchman, dedicated his hospital to the Holy Cross, alleged to have been discovered at Jerusalem by Helena, the mother of Constantine, and the Knights of St. John were both Hospitallers and Crusaders. Were they not the proper custodians ? Yet the vestiges of that pristine ideal are significant, though slight. The

---

[1] *Encyc. Brit.*, " Hy. de Blois."

Jerusalem, not the Maltese Cross, is the badge of the de Blois men, and is repeated on the buildings. Both have the equal limbs of the Greek as distinguished from the Latin Cross, both are eight-pointed, but the Maltese was a modification when, 400 years later, the Knights made their headquarters at Malta.

Intermittently, there arose scandalous abuses which did not wholly cease till 1851, when the case came before the Queen's Bench. William de Wykeham, who was created Bishop of Winchester in 1366, placed John de Campden as master of St. Cross, then despoiled and dilapidated, and he, serving it well for twenty-eight years, was buried before the high altar, where his memorial brass lies to this day.

Cardinal Beaufort (1377–1447) was the second son of John of Gaunt, and the successor of Wykeham. It was his intention to make a great addition to de Blois' foundation, and to him is given the credit of having so done. His " Hospital of Noble Poverty " was to provide *further* for two priests, thirty-five brethren and three nursing sisters, but he did not complete his plans, though his splendid gate-house suggests the scale of his design. In fact, the Wars of the Roses, in which the Yorkists were his enemies, Beaufort being naturally a Lancastrian, and the loss of his endowments, prevented him. It was left to his successor, Wayneflete, to fulfil his schemes, but he could only add, in his time, one priest and two brethren.[1]

Entering now the forecourt, on the east of which still stands the " Hundred Men's Hall," though long disused for its original purpose, we see before us Beau-

[1] *Vict. County Hist. of Hampshire.*

PLATE V.

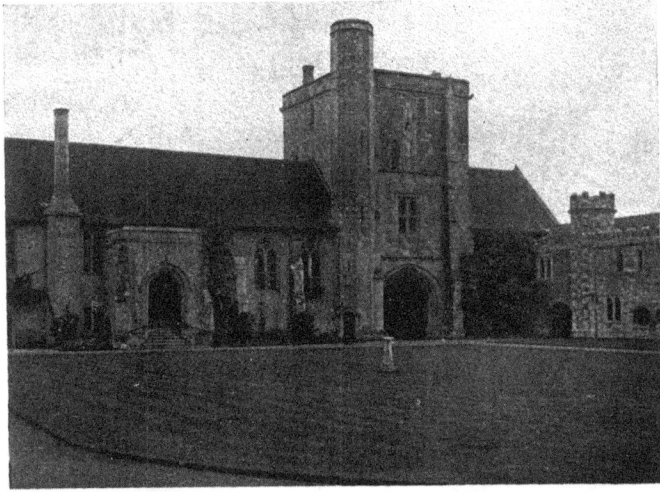

Fig. 6.--ST. CROSS, INNER COURT

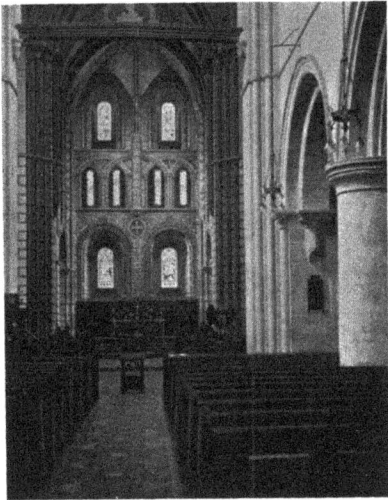

Fig. 7.—ST. CROSS, CHURCH

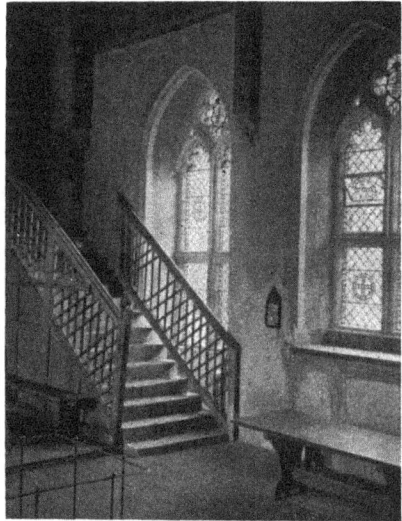

Fig. 8.—ST. CROSS, HALL

fort's towering gate-house, and through its archway a glimpse of that which lies beyond. Of the three canopied niches above the great window, which is that of the muniment room, one only contains a figure, that of Beaufort on his knees. The central and taller is said to have contained a representation of the Holy Cross, the third an effigy of de Blois. On the cornice of the second stage are carved heads, said to be those of John of Gaunt, Henry IV., Henry V., and Bishop Wykeham.[1] On the spandrils of the arch are, on the east, the royal arms, on the west, those of Beaufort, which are the same with a border for difference. On the south side of the tower a figure of the Virgin has been set up to replace that which fell about a hundred years ago.

The spacious inner court presents a verdant carpet of grass, with a sundial in its midst, while on west, north, and east are buildings, with the great church in the south-east. Walking round the lawn to the railings, which now bound open fields southwards, but where dwellings of the brethren formerly stood, and looking round, the impression is one of dignity and repose. (See Fig. 6.) Immediately to the left of the gate-house is the brethren's hall, or refectory, reached by ascending steps within a porch. On the west side are the tall chimneys and the entrances to the brethren's rooms, while similar chimneys are continued on the north, where formerly were brethren's chambers, and where later the master had his apartments. The master has now a house outside, but close to the hospital, with the general tone of which it accords, and the

[1] Sergeant's *Winchester*

brethren have been restored to the rooms from which they had long ago been ousted. On the east is a covered way known as the ambulatory or cloister. The upper storey was once the infirmary, and both parts are connected by an octagonal brick and stone turret on the north, while southwards they communicated with the north transept of the church. An inscription on an oriel about the centre shows the entire work of this part to have been that of Robert Sherborne, who was master in 1503, save the upper window, which was made by Henry Compton, D.D., master in 1667, and afterwards Bishop of London. It would seem to have been Compton who appropriated the brethren's rooms on the north side, at any rate his arms appear there, while Sherborne's motto—*dilexi sapientiam,* I have chosen wisdom—seen in rooms over the porter's lodge to the east of the gatehouse, suggests that these were the master's original quarters.

Each brother has a sitting-room, bedroom and kitchen to himself, and a portion of garden behind. The men of the de Blois foundation wear a black gown, a broad black cap, and the white Hospitallers' badge on the left breast, and at the present time they number 18. The Beaufort men, of whom there are 9, have a red gown of a fine deep shade, and a cardinal's hat as badge. It is only on special occasions that they dine in the refectory, yet it is a typical mediæval banqueting hall, with music gallery, "screens" below it, and central hearth. The windows are fourteenth century, but the corbels supporting the roof and some glass in the windows display the arms of Beaufort. The dimensions are

45 feet by 25. Both Miss Clay and Sidney Heath give good drawings of it, and it may be stated that the stairs shown in Fig. 8 lead to the muniment room in the gate-house.

Directly one enters the Church the impression is that of a noble Norman fane, while the massive pillars of the nave might suggest an early phase of the style. Yet there is nothing to meet the eye earlier than the mid-twelfth century ; in fact, the writer in the Victoria County History of Hampshire dates the work of the choir and the easternmost bay of the nave as 1160–1200. The influence from the Orient had already led to a real renaissance which gradually developed into the quite different grace of the Early English, and in this church we actually see the passage of the round-headed to the pointed arch. While the early windows are round, or one-centred, the vaulting throughout is pointed, or two-centred, as are all the supporting arches. Looking eastward down the nave one is struck with its loftiness, terminating with the three tiers of windows and the beauty of the interlacing arches of the triforium. The apparent square heads of the middle tier of windows is caused by partial external blocking. " Engaged " shafts, clustered or single, and in many places thrusting their delicate forms high aloft, are all capped with typical transition Norman carving. It is interesting to notice that the thirteenth century builders, in continuing the work of those who built before them, did not markedly depart from the original design, the massive columns being extended to the west end of the nave. One might wish to see less of the prevailing chevron or zigzag ornament, and more of the varieties

E

used by the Norman builders, nevertheless, there are pleasing effects of the chevron, as where two lines of it enclose lozenge-shaped spaces, sometimes in themselves decorated, while in one window of the north transept the outermost voussoirs, or arch-stones, each display a bird's head with a long beak pointing inwards, and the carving of the nave capital seen in Fig. 7 produces ornament often witnessed in other churches of the same period. Butterfield was a distinguished Victorian architect who restored the church about 1870, and he it was who painted the masonry of the choir. Although the " old men " did indeed paint their churches, partly for decoration, partly for instruction, and though some modern architects employ colour in their interiors, the question arises whether this is not like " painting the lily." There were, as has been indicated, later extensions and additions in the thirteenth and the following centuries, such as the Early English west door and window, the clerestories and the perpendicular stone screens on north and south of the choir. Indeed, there is evidence that the vaulting was not quite finished till Beaufort's time, for his arms appear on parts of it. Westward of the screen on the north of the choir is some wood-carving of the Tudor period, evidently the top of a screen, while similar work, somewhat patched together, is now suspended in the south choir aisle.

Sir Arthur Quiller-Couch has written a book, " Brother Copas," 1911, based on St. Cross and Winchester. With admirable light touch, he depicts in purely imaginative manner the life of the old place as it might be in the present day. The dear old master, gentleman and scholar, might be the Edward Burton of Whitgift's Hospital ledger book, or the present writer's fancied portrayal of him elsewhere. " Q " writes with intimate knowledge of " St. Hospital " and " Merchester," and his picture of the master's sunset walk through his domain is perfect.

SUSSEX

Chichester.—As we should expect, this cathedral city has its house of pity. In a side street, near the beautiful early sixteenth-century cross, is an unassuming little building known as St. Mary's Hospital, yet within we shall discover a gem of that most artistic age, the thirteenth-fourteenth centuries. Originally founded in 1172 as a convent for nuns by William, dean of the cathedral, it was re-constituted in the time of Henry III. for a master and thirteen poor men who had permanent quarters and provided as well for the sick and wayfarers. An extract from the statutes reads as follows : " If any one in infirm health and destitute of friends should seek admission for a term until he shall recover, let him be gladly received and assigned a bed. . . In regard to the poor men who are received late at night and go forth in the morning, let the Warden take care that their feet are washed and, as far as possible, their necessities attended to." At the present time, St. Mary's provides for a master, who has his quarters by the entrance gate, and eight aged women, four, with two rooms each, on either side of the hall under its low-reaching roof. At the eastern end is the lovely chapel, the whole building being of the

" infirmary type," as St. John's, Northampton, and Chiceley's bede-house at Higham Ferrers (pp. 31 and 32). The chimneys and wooden rails in the hall are of much later date, as is seen by an inscription.

Arundel.—It is interesting to find that this place, overlooking the gorge of the river Arun, had its hospital in the fourteenth century. An old writer, Dallaway, called it " Domus eleemosynaria," and said it was founded in his day by Richard, third Earl of Arundel, about 1380, for twenty-four poor, aged and feeble men who were not allowed to marry or re-marry on pain of expulsion, the master being an ecclesiastic. It survived till the Dissolution, and the buildings lasted till the Civil War of the seventeenth century.

Lewes.—There were two hospitals in this ancient county town of Sussex, placed at the northern foot of the South Downs, just where the river Ouse has carved its way through, and defended of old by the castle of the de Warrens at the summit of the pass. St. James', near the gate of the former Cluniac Priory, was for thirteen poor brethren and sisters. St. Nicholas' is said to have been erected by the founder of the Priory and also provided for thirteen poor brethren and sisters.

East Grinstead.—In this town, on the northern border of Sussex, where it adjoins the eastern part of Surrey, is Sackville College, a picturesque range of buildings with forecourt and outer gate-house, established under the will of Robert Sackville, second Earl of Dorset. Robert, himself an able man, was the son of Thomas, the first earl of this family, High Treasurer to Elizabeth and James I., who was not only a

PLATE VI.

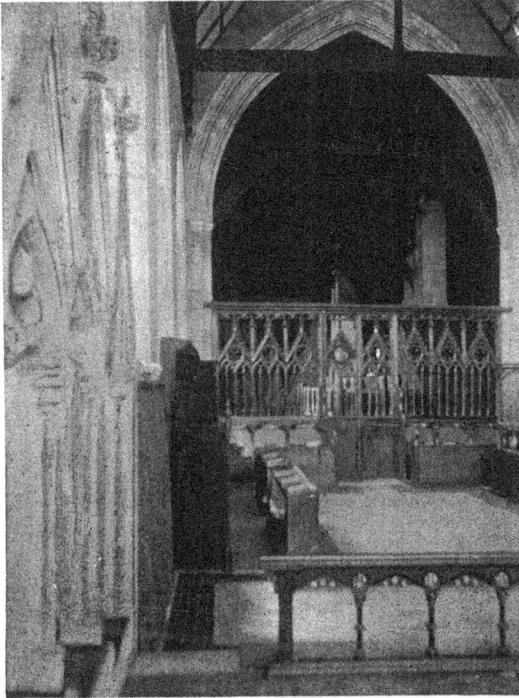

Fig. 9.—ST. MARY'S, CHICHESTER

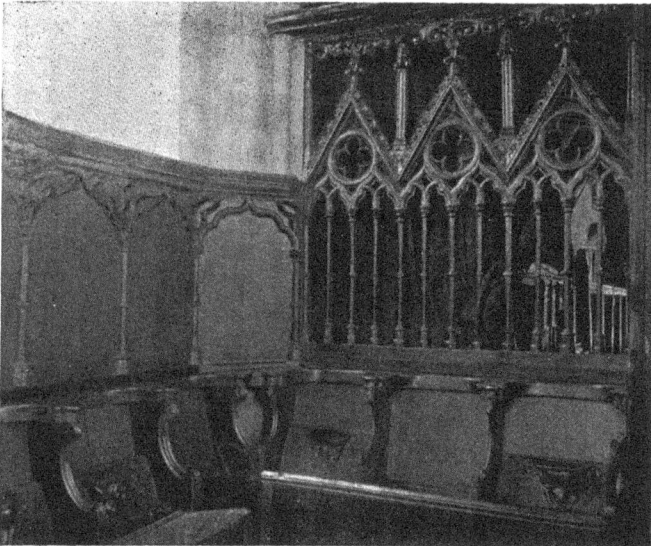

Fig. 10.—ST. MARY'S, DETAILS

[*Face p. 56*

distinguished statesman but a very notable man of
letters.   Robert's intentions were to provide for twenty-
one single and unmarried men and ten women, but,
dying in 1609, he had to leave to his executors what
they were never able to fully carry out.   The hospital
or college does not appear to have been opened before
1619—ten years after the founder's death—and the
third earl is stated to have completed it in 1622.   The
Act of Parliament for establishment did not pass till
1624, while the charter of incorporation was not
granted till 1631.   All this delay seems to have been due
to the unsatisfactory state of Robert Sackville's estates
at his death, encumbrances and entails creating un-
certainties and consequent long-drawn litigation, during
which the poor pensioners were reduced to a pitiable
state, some even dying of starvation.   When at length,
in 1700, the business was settled, the income of £300 a
year which the founder willed for his poor people was
reduced to £217.   At present there are eighteen inmates—seven women with rooms and £14 pension, four
men with the same, and seven women with rooms only.
By the founder's statutes, the warden is appointed by
his heirs, with residence and £28 per annum, and there
were two assistant wardens chosen from the persons of
standing in the town.   Some of the wardens were at
first pensioners, but others were men of distinction.   One
warden (1646–56) was a parson, and kept a grammar-
school, in which a future Bishop of Bath and Wells
was a pupil.   John Mason Neale was warden in 1846.
He was D.D., a distinguished ecclesiastical historian,
and a poet.   Partly at his own expense, he caused a
restoration of the buildings, and appears to have had

the independence to continue his services in the chapel, to which, indeed, the founder's statutes directed him, although the Bishop of Chichester inhibited him for thirteen years. Neale's exertions also led to the establishment of St. Margaret's Home.

CHAPTER VII

More West Saxon Shires

Berkshire, the ancient Berroc (box-tree) scir, takes its peculiar shape from skirting the right bank of the winding Thames, which everywhere bounds it north-wards, first as far as Oxford, and then flowing on, past Old Windsor Park at the eastern point of the county, continues its course and divides Surrey from Middlesex. In its southern part, Berkshire is dominated by the far-reaching chalk range which presents on its northern face the " Great Escarpment " of the geologists, save where its smaller eastern portion merges into the pine-clad heaths of Surrey. Between Walling-ford northwards and Reading southwards, the Thames has, in ages long passed, carved its course through the chalk, while, all the way from Oxford to Windsor, it yields a long succession of lovely river-scenes for our delight.

Far to the west of the county, the Downs reach a height of 856 feet in Whitehorse Hill, where, on the steep slope near its summit, the famous " White Horse," a rude figure 374 feet long, kept there perenially by removal of the turf from the chalk beneath, has been displayed since the un-historic past. The Vale of White Horse, as a broad geographical term, might be said to embrace all the land between the Berkshire Downs and the Cotswolds of Gloucestershire, but, in

the restricted sense usually adopted, it applies to the
much smaller area through which the little river Ock
flows eastwards to its junction with the Thames.
Perhaps, as the late T. W. Shore suggested, this district
was settled by the Frisian tribe of Hockings who gave
their name to the small river and to the not far-distant
crossing of the larger one at Oxford.[1]   This land and
its people are charmingly depicted in Eleanor Hayden's
" Islands of the Vale."   All that portion of the county
which lies north of the Downs is but slightly undulating
and is given over to agriculture.

Historically, Berkshire is distinguished above all
other counties by its special association with the
Kings of England.   First and uniquely, in the centre
of the market-place of Wantage, stands the statue of
England's greatest and most noble king—Alfred ; for
here he was born in 849.   Wantage, a little country
town nigh to the foot of the chalk downs, is further
distinguished in having a noble cruciform church, mainly
of thirteenth century date, the many carved and varied
corbels which support its roof adding interesting features
to the fabric.   Next and more conspicuously, Windsor
Castle has been the historic chief home of the Kings and
Queens of England ever since the Norman Conquest.

Reading, the county town, was once famous for the
great and powerful Benedictine Abbey, its mitred abbot,
it is said, taking precedence only after those of Glastonbury and St. Alban's.   In a dark and illiterate age, the
Conqueror's youngest son, styled for his comparative
learning Henry Beauclerc, founded and endowed the
abbey and was buried there.   His monument remained

[1] *Origin of the Anglo-Saxon Race.*

before the high altar, was repaired by order of Richard II., and was undisturbed till it was desecrated by a later age. At the Dissolution, Hugh Cook, who appears to have been the last abbot, from his name being at the end of the list given in *Monasticon*, willingly surrendered, but was nevertheless hanged and quartered for denying the King's supremacy. Thereafter, in lamentable ignorance of the beauties of architecture, the roof was treated as if it were a timber-yard and the walls a quarry, in order to build a new church and other places. The arms of the abbey were *Azure*, three escallops *Or*, and two seals are described in the British Museum Catalogue as of the twelfth and fourteenth centuries. Several parliaments were held at Reading Abbey, from Richard I. to Edward IV.

Three hospitals are mentioned in *Monasticon* as formerly existing at Reading. St. Lawrence was founded by Angerus, second abbot, before 1134, for twenty-six poor people, and the entertainment of strangers and pilgrims : the seal showed a bishop with mitre and staff, but no legend. St. Mary Magdalene's was a lazar-house outside the Abbey's gate and founded by Hugh, eighth abbot, about 1190, for twelve lepers. A third hospital was attached to the abbey, for widows of poor townsmen. These had to take vows of celibacy and " serve God day and night," praying for the king and the souls of founder and benefactors. The funds were misappropriated by an abbot, and were eventually used for establishing the grammar-school, at which Archbishop Laud was a scholar and became a considerable benefactor. St. Mary's came to nothing through the misappropriation of Abbot Thorne in the time of Edward IV., while St. Lawrence also perished, probably with the Abbey.

At Newbury St. Bartholomew's Hospital is said to have been founded by King John, who granted a fair upon St. Bartholomew's Day. Queen Elizabeth vested it by charter in the Corporation of Newbury. *It is still known* as King John's Court, and supported in 1830 six male and six female pensioners.

At Lambourn is a hospital founded by John Isbury towards the end of fifteenth or early in the sixteenth century for ten poor men, six being nominated by New College, Oxford, and four by the family of Hippesley in Lambourn. According to *Monasticon*, its continuation was secured by Act of Parliament in 31st Elizabeth, the ten men therein receiving in 1830 22s. per week, three loads of wood, and a portion of wheat and malt yearly, with a share of the fine paid every year for renewing of the lease. " Yet in being " are its words.

Abingdon, like Reading, had its great abbey, which existed from the seventh century and had, at the date of *Domesday*, possessions less extensive only than those of the Crown. Henry I. was placed there to be educated. That which remains from the Dissolution is limited to the guest-house, a beautiful gateway, ruins of the " prior's house," and other fragments.

The hospital of St. Helen was founded by Geffrey Barbar and John de Helen in the reign of Henry V. Leland, who began his itinerary before the Dissolution, speaks of six men and the same number of women being maintained there by the Guild of Holy Cross, whose functions were, besides the building of bridges and the repairing of highways, the maintenance of poor people.

The hospital was dissolved with the chantries, but refounded in 1553 by Sir John Mason, with the support of Edward VI., under the name of **Christ's Hospital,** for thirteen poor men and women. The parish church of St. Helen, Abingdon, is remarkable for its lofty north tower and steeple, and as having double aisles to its nave, each portion receiving a separate name or dedication. Its close connection with the ancient foundations is witnessed by the fact of a *parvise* in the tower having of old time been the exchequer chamber of the Fraternity of Holy Cross and, till lately, the muniment room of Christ's Hospital. Furthermore, all the buildings. both old and newer, are within the precincts of the church. And yet, save for one more recent addition, there is no religious limitation to admissions. The oldest portion stands apart on the west side of the churchyard.

The workmanship of the little round-headed arches of the fronting corridor is evidently the very latest in the perpendicular style, while the entrance porch is Elizabethan or Jacobean. There are some quaint coloured drawings under glass in its front, and texts from Scripture. Behind the corridor, which runs the whole length of the building, are the inmates' rooms and the little hall, while in the rear is a large garden with turf and curiously clipped yew bushes. The members of the sixteenth-century foundation consist of fourteen men and women. The hall has a bay window towards the garden with heraldic glass, is wainscoted to the ceiling in small oak panels with fine mouldings, and contains the contemporary portraits of Edward VI. and Sir John Mason.

East Hendred.—In this quaint little Berkshire village is the long desecrated but now restored chapel of Jesus of Bethlehem. It was built by the Carthusians of Sheen (Richmond), who established a cell in this parish in the fifteenth century. A screen entirely divides the western part from the sacrarium, thus forming the half upper storey into a loft or gallery, while both floors have separate doors into an adjoining but considerably later building called the priest's house. What purpose these small buildings served, in their present form, is obscure, for they stand a little apart, at the junction of three roads, from the remnant of the monks' house. Mr. Philip Palmer, master of Abbot's Hospital, Guildford, thinks it was a road-side hospital, and so it might have become after the so-called priest's house was attached. This is also in two stories, and might have accommodated both men and women, whether they were sick, wayfarers, or pilgrims. Yet the present writer is inclined to think that originally the chapel stood alone, without loft or adjoining house, purely as an oratory served by a priest from the Carthusian cell, where, perchance, a passer-by might " snatch an early mass."[1]

In Parker's work, where this little structure and certain domestic chapels are described and illustrated,[2] there is mention of Wiggeston's Hospital, Leicester, where the lower floor communicates directly with the chapel and the upper overlooks it as from a gallery, the only separation being a screen. In this connection

[1] EDWARD BRUCE : " I chanced, at early dawn, to pass
The chapel gate to snatch a mass."
—Scott's *Lord of the Isles*, Canto V., 9.
[2] *Ancient Domestic Architecture.*

it is instructive to notice the chapel at Ripley, although it is in Surrey.

Ripley Chapel.—In the Bishop of Winchester's Register it is stated that Ruald de Calva, in 1321, gave the church of Send, in Surrey, and the " Oratory of Ripeli " to the Priory of Newark. In the report of Edward VI.'s Commissioners " to enquire after Chauntries," Ripley is mentioned again, as a chapel of ease to the parish of Send, and as " builded long time past for an Hospital and sithen altered." It is uncertain if there ever was an *ancient* nave to this little church, but the present chancel is a beautiful example of transition Norman. The finely-carved vaulting shafts support nothing, and it is evident that the original design of the builders was never carried out. " Oratory " in the words of the fourteenth-century donors seems to imply that it was *at that time* a chapel of ease to Send, while those of Edward's Commissioners suggest that at some *unknown date* it ceased for a time to have that function and became a hospital, reverting later to its original purpose. This may explain the absence of vaulting.[1]

Donnington, Berks.—Leland states that Sir Thomas Chaucer, son (or possibly nephew) of the poet, was the founder of a hospital in this place, while Dugdale says that William de la Pole, Duke of Suffolk, who married Sir Thomas' daughter, as will be more fully dealt with in Chapter VIII., is to receive the credit. Dugdale's editors, however, found the Patent Rolls giving an earlier date, namely, 1393, and Sir Richard Atterbury

[1] See illustrated article by P. M. Johnston, F.S.A., in *Surrey Arch. Colls.*, Vol. XVI.

as the founder of a house for thirteen poor men, one over them being described as the " minister of God of the Poor House at Donnington." After the Dissolution, Charles Howard, Earl of Nottingham, the Lord Howard of Effingham of Armada fame, petitioned Queen Elizabeth for restoration of the estates, which had remained in the Crown till 1570. Howard completed Atterbury's foundation, and his statutes controlled the hospital *as late, at least, as* 1830.

Lyford, in the Vale of White Horse, is a tiny village set in the midst of cornfields and pasture. By the side of a lane which leads to the parish church and adjoining manor-house are brick piers and gates. Passing through, one enters straightway the little place depicted in Fig. 11. These are the almshouses founded by Oliver Ayshcombe, 1610, whose family then held the manor, for deserving persons of Lyford, East, and West Hanney. Note the little pent-houses over each door —they are numbered from 1 to 20—the chapel in the centre of the further side, and the pump. There is a large garden in the rear. The inmates, who must be over 60 years of age, (and men's wives, if any, are now admitted as separate pensioners) receive their presentation at the hands of the trustees. The place is delightfully described by Miss Hayden.

" The Vicar of Bray " used to be a favourite song in the writer's student days. The ballad is traditionally ascribed to a trooper in the reign of George I., and tells how a man " turned his coat " through successive political changes and still held on to his benefice. Who was the prototype (if any) is uncertain, but one, Simon Aleyn, was vicar from *c.* 1540 to 1588, and had the reputation of being alternately Protestant and Papist.[1] The village is beautifully situated on the chalk by the right bank of the Thames, a little south of Maidenhead. Here we find Jesus Hospital, founded by William Goddard in 1609, under the control of the Fishmongers' Company, for the six most aged freemen and freewomen of the company, thirty-four from the poorest parishioners of Bray who have been resident for twenty years and not less than 50 years old. The rooms are arranged around a quadrangle, and, besides the chapel, there are a common kitchen and bakehouse. This place, with its warm red brick and its green court, is said to be the prototype of Frederick Walker's celebrated " Harbour of Refuge."[2]

Buckinghamshire is, geographically, separated wholly from Berkshire, but geologically it is one with it and Oxfordshire. The chalk range, known as the Chilterns beyond Reading, passes through the southern part of the county in a north-easterly direction, rising to 900 feet. There are no outstanding ecclesiastical or historical associations attaching to the county, but these immortal names cling to it—John Hampden, Edmund Burke, John Milton, and Gray, whose " Elegy in a Country Churchyard" centres round the "ivy-mantled tower " of Stoke Poges, which the present writer has never yet seen, though Americans, at any rate, make pilgrimage thither.

In High Wycombe is the hospital of St. John the Baptist, founded by some person unknown, about 1180, for a master, brethren and sisters. Late Norman

[1] *Encyc. Brit.*
[2] Sidney Heath, *op. cit.*

remains are seen in the hall, and a fair was established for its benefit. In 1334 it was under the patronage of the mayor and burgesses, and *is still in the charge of the town*, Queen Elizabeth having refounded it after the Dissolution.

At Newport Pagnell a hospital, dedicated to St. John the Evangelist and St. John the Baptist, was founded about 1281 by John de Somery. It was refounded by Anne, queen of James I., for three poor men and three poor women above 50 years of age, the Vicar of Newport Pagnell being *ex officio* master. *It still exists.*

OXFORDSHIRE

Oxford.—Tanner records St. Bartholomew's, within half a mile east of the city, as existing in his time. It was a small hospital founded by Henry I. for a master, two " healthful " brethren, and six infirm or leprous brethren. Being of royal foundation, Edward III. gave it to Oriel College, Oxford, which had to maintain it. *It still exists* near Cowley Marsh. " The Hospital of St. John, without the East Gate of Oxford, consisting of a master and several brothers and sisters, was in being in the reign of King John [1209], who was a benefactor to it. King Henry III. new-founded, or at least new-built it, A.D. 1233, laying the first stone himself. King Henry the Sixth gave the master and brethren leave to give up and convey this House and all the estates belonging to it to William Wainflet, Bishop of Winchester, about A.D. 1456, who on or near the site of it laid the foundation of his magnificent

College, with the Hall adjoining, to the honour of St. Mary Magdalene."—Tanner, quoted in *Monasticon*. " The building itself [of the ancient hospital] was but low, having the river Cherwell running under the east side of it ; and the Fabrick, according to those times, indifferent, part of which is yet standing, viz., the kitchen belonging to Magdalen College, the Divinity Reader's Lodgings, and the Chapel on the South side." John Peshall wrote thus in 1773, and is quoted in *Monasticon*, wherein it is stated that the seal still exists and bears an eagle surmounting a cross, the inscription being (Anglicised) " Common seal of the hospital house of St. John the Baptist beyond the east gate of Oxford." The hospital at Ewelme is also in Oxfordshire, but it deserves and shall have a chapter to itself.

F

CHAPTER VIII

The Hospital at Ewelme

It is pleasing, amidst records of robbery, misdirection of founder's purpose, and destruction, to deal with one place where none of these things have happened.

Nestling among the chalk uplands of Oxfordshire is the little village of Ewelme. Chalk springs issue here, and have probably given name to the place, *awl* being one of the many variants of a root-word signifying water.

The Founders.—William de la Pole, a faithful servant of Henry VI. and Margaret of Anjou, his queen, was created Duke of Suffolk and became the second husband of Alice Chaucer. She was the daughter of Sir Thomas Chaucer, whose name we have already met in connection with Donnington in Berkshire. It is certain that he succeeded England's first great poet, Geoffrey Chaucer, in one of his crown offices, but documentary evidence that he was a son or nephew is wanting. Alice, however, inherited both wealth and position, and brought her husband the Manor of Ewelme. As shown by his will, dated 1448, in which he mentions the God's-house at Ewelme, the Duke and his wife had already built their church and almshouse.[1]

Suffolk was treacherously murdered in 1450, and his

---

[1] Both Miss Clay and Sidney Heath give the date as 1437, but Dodd puts the completion of the chapel, which is also the parish church, at *c.* 1434.

mutilated body buried in a nameless grave in his ancestral church at Wingfield, Suffolk. The Duchess survived him till 1475, and on her tomb in Ewelme Church she alone is described as the founder. This apparent disloyalty to husband and father is probably to be attributed to the political disturbances of the times, which we have already seen as preventing the fulfilment of the great Cardinal's plans at St. Cross. Under normal conditions, the widow would have set up a monument to her husband and herself during her own lifetime, leaving a space for recording the day of her death. But to have done so shortly after the Duke's death might have displeased the rival house of York. To have placed an inscription on the tomb at Wingfield might have been unacceptable to Henry's Court, who probably feared the popular feeling against Suffolk for his diplomacy, which led to the surrender of Anjou and Maine to France, and who did nothing to bring his murderers to justice. Anyhow, the Duchess transferred her allegiance to the opposite side, and married her son John to a daughter of Richard, Duke of York. It was this Duke John who erected the monument to his mother.

The Almshouse.—Ascending a slight elevation, let us enter Ewelme Almshouse, as it is generally called, by the outer gate and thence, by a doorway from the forecourt, the rustic cloisters which surround on all sides a little square inner court 36 feet wide. Opening on to the cloisters are the thirteen brethren's living rooms (the original number) set in herring-bone brickwork between oaken framing, while in the roofs appear the dormer windows of their bedrooms. In the centre of each side of the cloisters an open porch with lovely bargeboard gives access from the court, and steps behind the east side lead up to a covered way into the western tower of the church, through a richly-carved and moulded doorway. All within this beautiful edifice is *perpendicular at its best*, and unaltered. There is no chancel arch, but a fine screen, mainly of carved wood, divides off the eastern portion, and by its extension north and south separates its aisles from those of the nave. J. A. Dodd, M.A., tells us that the chancel screen formerly supported a rood-loft, approached by steps outside the north wall. The south chancel aisle is dedicated to St. John the Baptist, and has a beautiful panelled roof. Here is the altar-tomb of Thomas Chaucer, with brass effigies of himself and his wife. Here also are the seats allotted to the brethren with one in the centre for the master, and all are backed with high wainscot moulding. Between the eastern end of St. John's chapel and the sanctuary is the most notable feature of the church, to wit, the monument to the Duchess. This is minutely described by Mr. Dodd in a valuable little book, which can be purchased by visitors to Ewelme. It is to be noted that Alice de la Pole wears the Garter ribbon on her left arm, a privilege granted to very few women, and through the open tracery below is seen an obscure dark object. This represents the body of the Duchess wrapped in cerements of the grave, a remarkable but by no means uncommon accompaniment of the splendour above, not only here but[1] especially in the eastern counties.

---

[1] I am told by Mr. R. R. Hutchinson, of Wallingford, that the addition of shrouded figures came into practice about the fifteenth century, and lasted through Tudor times. He also cites the tomb of Archbishop Chiceley in

PLATE VII.

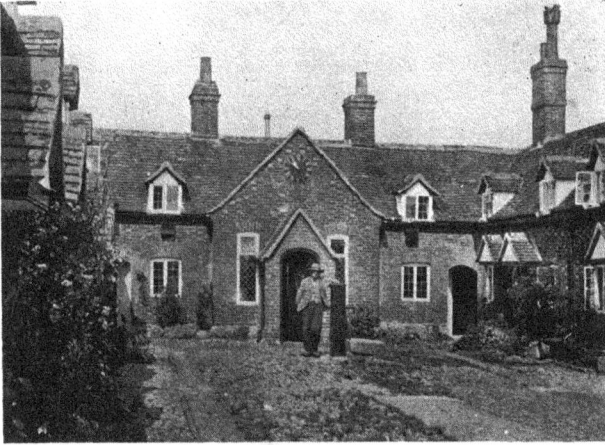

Fig. 11.—ALMSHOUSES, LYFORD, BERKS

(*See p. 66*)

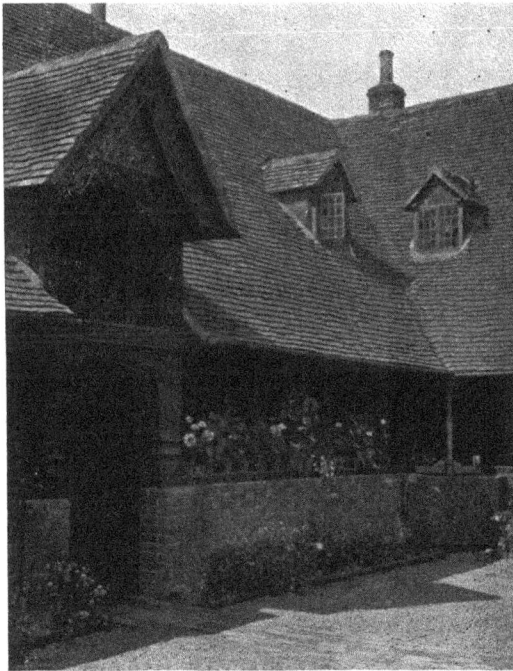

Fig. 12.—EWELME, ALMSHOUSE

[*Face p. 72*

An interesting illustration of this East Anglian influence is given by the Rev. J. E. Field. This writer says that Ewelme Church is unlike the Oxfordshire churches, but is "modelled upon that which Michael, the first Earl, built at his home at Wingfield." This Michael, descended from the wealthy mercantile family of atte Pole in Hull, was created Earl of Suffolk in 1385. He acquired Wingfield through marriage, in addition to his estates in Yorkshire and Lincolnshire.

Provisions and Statutes of the Founders.—Having seen together this beautiful and lively memorial of the benevolent founders, let us glance at their statutes so that we can the better understand how it escaped unscathed the hands of the destroyers. The endowment was ample for thirteen poor men and two chaplains, one to be master of the house and, if possible, a "degreed" man. The other chaplain was to be master of the free school adjoining, which still remains. The founders insist upon visitation by their representatives, and provide that the Lord Chancellor of England shall be the protector of the revenues. Besides some pious observations regarding themselves and their beneficiaries, in which we hear an echo from Henry de Blois of three hundred years before, the founders enact certain stringent regulations for master and poor men. There were frequent services, as in a monastery, and the bedesmen had to repeat a bidding prayer around the founders' tombs (this in ignorance of the duke's future burial elsewhere), for King Henry VI., the Duke and

Canterbury Cathedral where it occurs. In the Chantry of Bishop Fox in Winchester is a like arrangement. I have seen one of these gruesome effigies by itself in Sanderstead Church, Surrey.—J. M. H.

Duchess of Suffolk, their parents, and all Christian souls. The bedesmen's garb was a tabard with a red cross on the breast, and a hood in accordance. The inmates were a corporation with a common seal. As for the master, he was to be one who could counsel the poor men and was to omit none of the services, not even " for pleasure of lord or lady," save " if he be let by sickness or preaching the word of God or by visitation of father or mother." There appear to have been no abuses during the following hundred years, so that there was nothing upon which Henry VIII.'s commission could found accusation, and the place, though in reality a chantry, remained unspoilt. The governance is still in private hands.

Further history of the de la Poles.—The family reached its zenith in respect to rank when Duke John married into the princely house of York. But its elevation was the occasion of its undoing. Of John's three sons, John, created Earl of Lincoln by Edward IV. during his father's lifetime, and nominated by Richard III. to the throne, died fighting against Henry VII. at Stoke-on-Trent, and his possessions, including those he would inherit on the death of his sire, were declared forfeited to the Crown. Edmund, the second son, though treated with clemency by Henry VII., who pardoned him of a murder, laid claim while in exile to the Crown of England. He was taken prisoner and finally beheaded without trial by Henry VIII. Richard, the third son, embarked on a futile invasion of England, was known in France as " La Blanche Rose," and fell fighting in the service of Francis I. in his expedition into Italy. Thus ended in 1525 the chequered history

PLATE VIII.

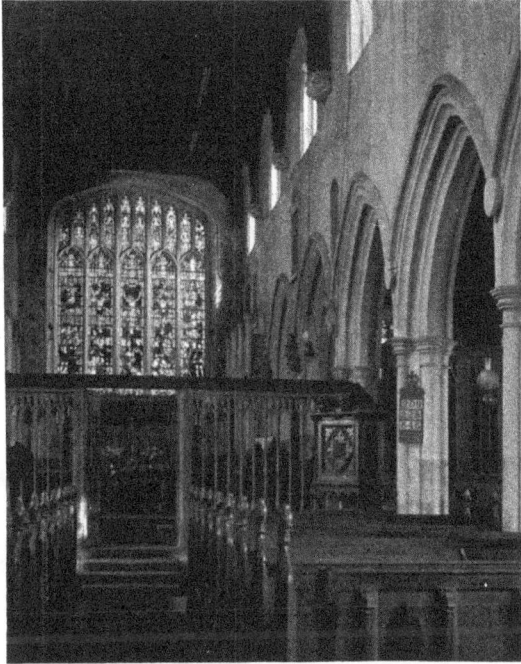

Fig. 13.—EWELME, CHAPEL

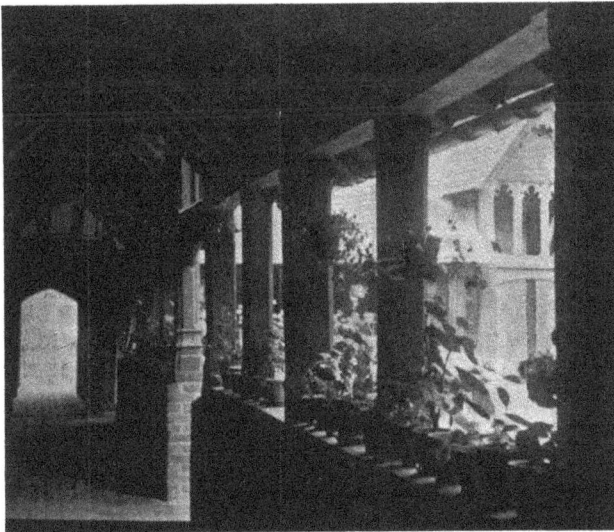

Fig. 14.—EWELME, CLOISTERS

of the Pole family, and so died the last male of the House of York.[1]

James I. annexed the mastership of the almshouse to the Regius Professorship of Medicine at Oxford, and so it remains.

[1] The history of the Pole family is in part taken from an article in the *Encyc. Brit.* by Oswald Barron, F.S.A.

CHAPTER IX

East Anglia

LINCOLNSHIRE

Historic Lincoln, British, Roman and Mediæval, has not retained one of its old hospitals, which appear to have been originally lazar-houses.

Tatershall had an almshouse attached to a college of the time of Henry VI. The site was granted by Henry VIII. to Charles Brandon, Duke of Suffolk, his brother-in-law and grandfather of Lady Jane Grey.

Spittel on the Street, in the same county, evidently derives its name from a hospital in the parish of Helmeswell, founded before 1323, and dedicated to St. Edmund. It was augmented by Thomas Aston, a canon of Lincoln in the time of Richard II., and was "*yet in being*" in 1830.

NORFOLK

King's Lynn.—Petrus Capellanus founded St. Mary Magdalene's in 1145 for a prior and twelve brethren and sisters, nine of whom were to be "sound" and three leprous. It flourished till the time of Edward VI., when it appears to have been disendowed, but not actually suppressed. It lingered on thence till refounded by James I., who re-endowed it with its ancient possessions. *In 1830* there were a master and eleven poor widows.

Norwich, unlike the sister city of Lincoln, was rich in ancient hospitals, several of which continue to the present day. In the time of Edward I., John le Grant founded a God's-house in St. Giles' parish. Later, Richard de Brockles refounded it as St. Saviour's, which King Edward confirmed in 1304. It is now extinct.

St. Paul's, called also Normanspital (Tanner) from Norman, its first master, was begun by the Prior and Convent of Norwich, and finished between 1121 and 1145. At first it was for men and women, but later for fourteen women, seven of whom were called " whole-sisters " and seven " half-sisters " of the Normans, under a master placed by the monks of the cathedral. After the Dissolution, the hospital was converted into a bridewell " for Lazy beggars " in 1571, and used as such under the corporation till 1785. The revenues were still applied in 1830 for St. Andrew's Bridewell, the remains of the hospital building being utilised for a malt-office.

St. Giles' was founded by Bishop Suffield, who in 1249 built the hospital and its church on a site purchased by him in Norwich. The first deed provided for four effective chaplains and all decrepit chaplains in the diocese, besides thirteen poor people who were to have one meal a day, evidently not as inmates. Suffield died in 1257, bequeathing 300 marks and his *gilt cap*, which had been the " Blessed St. Edmund's," etc. There were also considerable contemporary and later benefactions. In 1430 the constitution was a master, deacon, sub-deacon, eight chaplains, who wore the habit of Austin canons regular, seven scholars or choir-boys, four sisters, and eight poor bed-ridden people. Succour was given to travellers and pilgrims and other needy also. Though Henry VIII. intended the dissolution of the house, it was not till Edward VI.'s time that it was ecclesiastically dissolved, and then granted to the corporation. In 1821 the revenues were stated at £4,000, and there were 53 male inmates and 49 female. In 1830 an addition was erected for 24 more indigent people. *The hospital was then known as St. Helen's*, the ancient church being used for wards, and the beautiful roof of the choir, carved and gilded, in excellent preservation. It is still spoken of as St. Giles', or the old men's hospital. The seal is engraved in Blomefield's *History of Norfolk*, and is described in the British Museum catalogue in the following terms : " Late thirteenth century seal of the master and brethren : St. Giles seated on a throne with a fawn [hart] wounded by an arrow leaping up to him : on the left a tree : in the base, under a round-headed arch, a cross surmounted by a mitre." (See Chap. II., p. 11).

There were, besides, at least eight other hospitals in Norwich, only *two or three of which now exist*.

Ivy Hall, sometimes called St. Mary's, was more often known in olden time as Hildebrond's, after a mercer of the city who founded it early in the thirteenth century, the patronage being in the hands of the bishop. The *Victoria History* gives an Anglicised extract from fourteenth century register of the archdeaconry, which says—" In which said hospital poor people *ought* to be entertained and to have a certain quantity of fuel from

the master." The writer then goes on to remark—
" The common fate of so many of these hospitals over-
took the one founded by citizen Hildebrond, namely,
the absorption of the major part of the income by the
master." This, indeed, happened too often in these
" religious " houses, where the advowson is often
mentioned as a valuable gift in the hands of great people,
putting it within the power of a dishonest incumbent
to enrich himself at the expense of the inmates, the poor
and helpless, their care, ostensibly the prime object of
the founder, being counted by those who were put in
trust but a troublesome and negligible annex. And
yet Hildebrond's somehow managed to pursue its
chequered career, and is mentioned in *Monasticon* as a
continuation of the mediæval foundation under the
Corporation in 1830.

The *Victoria History* tells of six hospitals which were
originally lazar-houses without the city walls. The
most important was St. Mary Magdalene's. " Here,
again, the whole funds seem to have been absorbed by
the chaplain or master," the last being mentioned in
1530, but, as the *present officials* are spoken of, the
inference is that it survives in some form. Of the lesser
lazar-houses, one was outside each of the principal gates
of the city. That dedicated to St. Mary and St. Clement
was outside St. Austin's gate, and is mentioned by
Tanner as existing in his time for the reception of poor
diseased persons, and known as the " Pest house."
St. Benedict's continued long after the Dissolution as a
poor-house ; St. Stephen's likewise as a hospital ;
another was probably dedicated to St. Leonard; and a
fifth was outside Newport or St. Giles' gate.

Thetford, in the south-west of the county and on the border of Suffolk, is a small market-town, but has the distinction of having been the original seat of the East Anglian bishopric, whence Bishop Herbert de Lozinga removed it to Norwich in 1096. No vestiges of the six ancient hospitals of Thetford now exist, but in the time of Francis Blomefield (1705–52) who wrote the *History of Norfolk* aforesaid, the hospital of St. Mary and St. Julian, as distinct from its chapel, was still standing. It was sometimes called " The Hermitage of St. Julian," and entertained poor travellers and pilgrims.[1]

SUFFOLK

Bury St. Edmunds.—The borough of St. Edmund, the Anglo-Saxon king slain by the Danes in 903, was long before his time a royal town. There were six hospitals here. (1) St. John the Evangelist's without the south gate. (2) St. Nicholas', without the east gate, with a master and several brethren, the foundation being ascribed to one of the Abbots of the monastery. It occurs in records as early as 1223, and in 1281 was placed under the protection of the precentor. (3) St. Petronella's at the south gate. (4) St. Stephen's (Tanner's *Index Monasticus*). (5) St. Peter's without Risby Gate is said to have been founded by Abbot

---

[1] On Sunday, January 25th, 1925, Dr. Bertram Pollock, Bishop of Norwich, re-dedicated and preached from a stone throne attributed to Herbert de Lozinga. This throne rises 15 feet above the floor of the choir, an oaken stair has been constructed, and upon a silver plate is an inscription in Latin to this effect :—" Herbert, the first Bishop of Norwich, is believed, on his return from Rome, to have built this Throne. Eight hundred years afterwards it was repaired by Bertram, who reproduced his predecessor's Throne, but failed in his desire to reproduce his eminence, his piety and his repentance."—*Daily News.*

Anslem, Henry I.–Stephen, for poor priests and others when infirm and old or leprous and diseased. Originally it was under the sole management of the Abbey's almoner. In 1551 protection was granted to the " lazars " in it, though there could hardly have been many, if any, leprous at that time, and the owners became the trustees of a grammar school. (6) St. Saviour's, near the north gate, was founded about 1184 by the Abbot and Convent, though it was not finished till the time of King John. At first there were a warden, twelve chaplain-priests, six clerks, twelve poor " gentlemen," and twelve poor women. In the time of Edward I., the poor sisters were to be dismissed and their places taken by old and infirm priests. St. Saviour's was the most considerable of its kind in the town. The Parliament of 1446 was held in it, and there Humphrey, Duke of York, was murdered, the same year. As was to be expected, so ecclesiastic a house as this did not survive the Dissolution.

CHAPTER X

KENT AND ESSEX

KENT

Canterbury.—Although the Anglo-Saxon Archbishop Stigand was displaced at the Conquest by the Italian Lanfranc, Wulfstan, Bishop of Worcester, afterwards canonised, who founded in that city a hospital in 1085, as we have seen in Chapter IV., enjoyed the good-will of that noble-minded scholar, educationalist, ecclesiastic and statesman. Lanfranc had great influence with William the Conqueror, and some with his son, William Rufus, and when he died, in 1089, was universally lamented.[1] He founded, contemporaneously with Wulfstan, the hospital of St. John the Baptist at Canterbury, for a hundred poor and impotent men and women. The buildings were of stone, but the greater part were destroyed by a fire in the fourteenth century. Part of the chapel remains, and shows a round-headed doorway ornamented with chevron or zigzag, figured by Miss Clay. Mr. Sidney Heath also gives a charming drawing of the present gate-house, which appears to be of sixteenth-century date. Eadmer (c. 1060– c. 1124), a notable contemporary writer and a monk of Christchurch, Canterbury, described the hospital, which, he said, had ample grounds. At one time a proctor was

---

[1] *Encyc. Brit.,* " Lanfranc."

employed to collect money and other gifts for the hospital, pardons sold by him giving to *penitents* exemption from 30,000 paternosters and aves. Vestments of Bruges satin and fustian are mentioned, and ancient documents and utensils are preserved at the hospital. *It survives to the present day*, with a prior and eighteen brethren, the Archdeacon of Canterbury presenting.

The lepers' house at Harbledown has been described in the chapter on Lazar-houses. A third hospital, deriving its origin from Lanfranc, was attached to the Priory of St. Gregory, founded by him about the same time. It did *not* survive the Dissolution.[1] We may note in this connection that, as Miss Clay says, every cathedral city had, at one time or another, a hospital or hospitals, though they did not in all cases owe their origin to bishops, who were bound by their consecration vows to have special care for the poor.

Sandwich.—St. Bartholomew's was founded sometime before 1227. The beautiful Early English chapel contains the effigy of Sir Henry de Sandwich in chain armour. He was Lord Warden of the Cinque Ports and a later benefactor to the hospital. The original homes of the brethren and sisters have not been preserved, but those substituted *are set like a little village about the church.*

Thomas Rayling, clerk, William Swan, clerk, John Goddard and Richard Long founded the hospital of St. Thomas in the time of Richard II. for twelve poor persons, and it *still exists.*

Hythe.—Hamo, Bishop of Rochester, and the Com-

---

[1] *Monasticon.*

monality of the port of Hythe, founded St. Andrew's in the time of Edward III., for ten poor men and women. *It still exists*, and is known as St. Bartholomew's.

Sevenoaks.—In the time of Edward III. the hospital of St. John the Baptist was under the patronage of the Archbishop of Canterbury. William Sennocke, who had been exposed as an infant in the streets—hence his name—when he became Lord Mayor of London amplified the hospital in 1418 for twenty poor men and women, and founded a free school. Sir John Potkin liberally endowed the foundation, and the *school remains to this day*.

Dartford.—Henry VI., in 1453, licensed John Bamburgh, William Rothole, Roger Jones and Thomas Boost to found a hospital for five poor persons, to be called " The Trinitees Almes House in Dartford," with the vicar and churchwardens of Dartford as perpetual governors, and to be a corporate body. Although a charge being paid in 1553 is recorded in *Monasticon*, there appears to be no further record of this place. Wat Tyler's house is still shown in Dartford.

Dover.—St. Mary's Hospital, or the Maison Dieu, erected and endowed early in the reign of Henry III. by Hubert de Burgo for the relief of pilgrims and several poor people, is figured and described at some length by Miss Clay in her book, though it does not now exist.

Rochester.—The Spital of St. Katherine at Eastgate was founded by Symond Potyn in 1316 for poor men of the city, leprous or otherwise diseased, and is *still existing*. See " Sketches of Rochester," C. Phippen.

Strood.—Gilbert de Glanvill, Bishop of Rochester, early in the reign of Richard I., built and amply endowed a hospital, dedicated to the Virgin, for poor travellers and other necessitous persons. The revenues and *site* were settled by Henry VIII. on the " new erected " Dean and Chapter of Rochester.

Maidstone.—Pilgrimage was, as all know, a very important factor in mediæval religious life and " Cold-harbours," in the language of the south, and " Windy-arbours," in that of the north, were real houses of pity for poor pilgrims overtaken by darkness, cold or wind on their journeys to the various shrines. These temporary structures have all vanished, and left but their names to roads or places.

Archbishop Boniface built a hospital beside the river Medway in the year 1260 for poor travellers and pilgrims on their way to the shrine of St. Thomas the Martyr at Canterbury. Archbishop Courtney, in 1395, grafted upon this a college of secular clergy. This partly ruined pile forms a picturesque object above the river at Maidstone.

ESSEX

The ancient kingdom of the East Saxons is rich in historical and ecclesiastical memories ; its nobles took a leading part in securing Magna Charta ; 5,000 of its peasantry joined the insurrection of 1381, and men of Essex were strong on the side of the Parliament in the Civil War. Though little remains of its numerous religious houses, the nave of the abbey church at Waltham Holy Cross still testifies through its ornate Norman architecture to the pristine splendour of that

G

monastery, and here King Harold was buried. Neither has Essex much to tell us now of surviving houses of pity.

In Colchester, the county town, Endo, founder of St. John's Abbey, erected also and dedicated to St. Mary Magdalene a hospital for a master and leprous persons, and Richard I. granted a fair to it. James I. refounded the hospital in 1610 for five unmarried poor persons, and it *remains to this day.*

At Ilford, the Abbess and Convent of Barking dedicated a hospital to the Virgin and St. Thomas the Martyr, for thirteen poor or leprous people. One authority dates its foundation in the time of Stephen, another says Henry II.—Richard I. After the Dissolution, Elizabeth granted the property to Thomas Fanshaw, Remembrancer to the Exchequer, on condition that he appointed a master and provided for the lodgment and sustenance of six poor persons. It may, therefore, be said to be *still " in being."*

Walthamstow.—St. Mary's parish church is of the early fifteenth century, but is now of no architectural interest. Close to the churchyard, however, is a picturesque row of red-brick almshouses with a grammar school's original quarters in the upper storey, which, though now let off, the school having been transferred to new buildings in the High Street, bears an inscription on its wall recording the building by Sir George Monoux in 1527. In the centre, with projecting gable, formerly dwelt the schoolmaster; on the ground floor on either side are the homes of thirteen poor people, as at first. Sir George Monoux was a member of the Drapers' Company, Lord Mayor of London, and died in 1543.

He is credited with having built the tower and north aisle of the church, adapting its east end as his private chapel. Here he was buried, and his memorial brass displays the arms of his company.[1]

---

[1] *Greater London*, Walford, who gives a view as seen from the churchyard. *Hospitals and Almshouses of London*, published by the Underground Company.

CHAPTER XI

WHITGIFT'S HOSPITAL IN SURREY

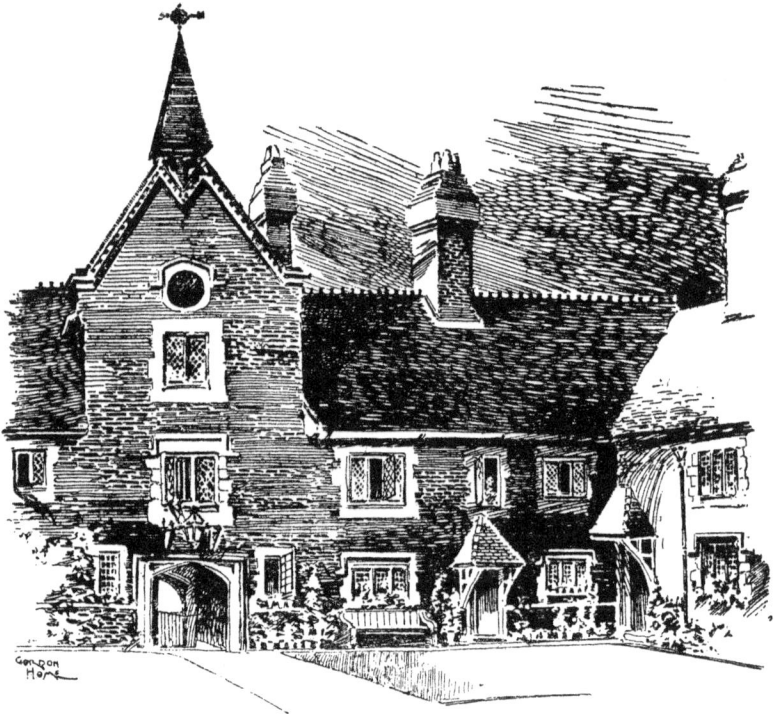

Fig. 15.—Whitgift's Hospital.
By permission of the Homeland Association.

JOHN WHITGIFT (1530-1604), a native of Great Grimsby in Lincolnshire, was the first Archbishop after Chicheley to found a hospital. The association of Croydon with the See of Canterbury was unbroken (unless we count the brief interval of the Commonwealth a break) from the ninth[1] to the close of the eighteenth century. Of the many rural manors belonging to the See, Croydon alone remained to it after certain " exchanges " between Henry VIII. and Archbishop Cranmer. The ancient manor-house of Croydon still exists as a secondary school under the Sisters of the Church at Kilburn, and is fully described in recent writings, such as the Victoria County History of Surrey and the Surrey Archæological Collections, Vol. XXIV., and in Ducarel's description,[2] where illustrations of the buildings are given as they were in the eighteenth century. It is frequently referred to in the archiepiscopal registers and letters from 1273 to 1752. Whitgift appears to have resided alternately at Lambeth and his country house of Croydon, to which he was the first to give the name of palace.[3] We find in this association Whitgift's choice of site and the almost exclusive selection of inmates from the parishes of Lambeth and Croydon.

This book is not the place wherein to discuss the ecclesiastical and political aspects of Whitgift's career ; it may be read in full in Strype's Life of the Archbishop, 3 vols., 1718, in Hooke's *Lives of the Archbishops*, and in the shorter and wholly laudatory memoir written by his friend and servant, Sir George Paule, 1612. What does concern us is to follow the development of his famous hospital during the latter years of a long and strenuously controversial life.

The first of the documentary stages was an enabling Act of Parliament in 1596, rendered necessary to give

[1] The late T. W. Shore discovered in the *Liber Aureus* a record of an exchange in 871. Dax Alfred had lands at Chartham in Kent, the Archbishop at Croydon.

[2] *Bibliotheca Topographica Britannica*, Vol. XII., 1783.

[3] *Chronicle of Croydon*, J. Corbet Anderson, 1882.

legal security for hospitals founded after the wholesale dissolutions of previous reigns. In this we may surmise the hand of Whitgift himself. The next takes the form of letters patent, dated November 22nd, the same year, authorising him to establish his hospital at Croydon and, at the "humble petition" of John Whitgift, nominating the first members, to wit, Elizabeth's "well beloved" Phillip Jenkins, as Custos or Warden, and the following six members (not called "well-beloved")—John Holland*, Christopher Fenner,* Reginald Scroobie,* Richard Dibble, Robert Curtis* and Thomas Whitehead. The third stage was Whitgift's Charter of Incorporation of 1599, the fourth a deed of gift, securing the property to the Warden and poor of the hospital for ever. We might add a fifth document, namely, Whitgift's Statutes and Ordinances, though they did not come fully into force during his life-time. They are to be seen in the Manuscript Library at Lambeth Palace, while the second, third, and fourth are preserved in Whitgift's Hospital. The statutes may also be obtained as a printed pamphlet. Elizabeth's letters form an interesting chart, illuminated, in Latin, engrossed on parchment, and having the Great Seal appended. The heraldry is characteristic of the age, and the royal claims to sovereignity not a little amusing. Elizabeth is styled "Regina Francie," where she had not one acre of land, while her possessions in the "Sister Isle" were deemed so unimportant as to be expressed by "Hibernie" in small letters. Whitgift's charter of incorporation has its own special interest. It is in English, also illuminated, signed "Jo Cantuar," and has his archiepiscopal seal attached. The document represents Whitgift holding the *corporate* seal in his hand, with the "history" of Dives and Lazarus, designed by himself and apparently unique, as already mentioned on p. 12. It again names Jenkins as warden and the first five brethren ; Whitehead's name has disappeared in the interval, but seven more are given, bringing the total to the traditional number of *thirteen*. These additional names are—Robert King, Edward Holloway, Edward Pringle,* Augustine Willis,* Henry Geoffrey,* Henry Leaver,* and Thomas Elton.*

The Deed of Gift is a tripartite indenture—note the actual *toothing* to tally with another part—is also in English and signed by George Whytgyft, the Archbishop's half-brother, and John Whitegift, his nephew, each spelling his name differently. Their private seals and the common seal of the hospital, without the warden's signature, are appended.[1] To read through either of these deeds would be a tedious task, though the late Warden, Alfred Jones, transcribed the whole of the Deed of Gift in his notes. Excerpts from the Charter (transcribed in full by Ducarel) are here given :—
" To all true Christian People to whom these presents shall come John Whitegift, Archbishop of Cant : primate of all England and metropolitan sendeth greeting in our Lord God Everlasting. . . Now this present deed witnesseth that the said J.W. archb : of Cant. . . . doth founde and establish the said

[1] The names marked with an asterisk, both in the Letters Patent and in the Charter of Incorporation, appear again among the admissions, though some not till 1604, the year of Whitgift's death, because up to that time they were in his service. The two other portions of the tripartite indenture were sealed respectively, by the Archbishop and the warden, and by the Archbishop and George and John Whitgift Junior.

building, or brickhouse . . . gardens, orchards, [etc.] to be an hospitall and abiding place for the finding, sustentation and relief of certain poore, needy or impotent people to have continuance for ever, which hospitall and the persons therein to be placed the said J.W. archb. of Cant. . . . hereby doth assigne limit and appointe to be incorporated, named and called by the name of The Hospitall of the Holye Trinity in Croydon of the foundation of J.W. Archb. of Cant: . . . And doth ordain . . . that the same hospitall shall consist of one Wardeine and of maymed poore and impotent persons not exceeding in all the number of forty which shall be the body and members of the said hospitall." The document then, after much more repetition, goes on to name and appoint the aforesaid warden and brethren. Whitgift, however, does not anywhere use the term " brother," but " poor," and no mention is made of school or schoolmaster.

Both these deeds of Whitgift have endorsements, and those on the deed of gift are as fresh as if written yesterday. They are, with those on the charter, here transcribed.

Endorsements on Charter of Incorporation.

Sealed and delivered in the presence of us

Ric : London	Jo : Bath and Wells
J. W. Fawkes	Thomas Nevile
Jhon Boys (steward)	John Parker
Ed. Aylworth	William Beestone
W. Barlow	Ed. Barker
ffrancis Butler	George Paule

Chr : Wormeall   Abraham Hartwell
John Gilpin   Richard Massinger
                         ffowlke Boughton

Willm Segar

Norroy King of Armes

(These signatures are given in *facsimile* by Ducarel.)

Endorsements on Deed of Gift.

Sealed and delivered the day and year first within written in presence of us
Ed. Aylworth
Abraham Hartwell
Michaël Murgatrod
Mathy Bradburie
Richard Massinger
ffowlke Boughton
Willm. Beestone
Thomas Eyton
William Barnes
Joseph Bull
William Gallamoure

22nd die Mense Augusti 1599 Estate and Seysine herupon taken by us
Ed. Aylworth
Abraham Hartwell
and delivered over to the within Named George Whitegift and John White-gift according to the auctoritie within men-tioned in the presence of
Michaël Murgatrod
Willm. Beestone
Samuell ffynche
Tho : Redman
Mathy Bradburie
ffrancis Butler

(The attached names are all autographs in the original.)

On January 17th, 1599, Whitgift, not waiting for Elizabeth's letters patent, began to prepare his ground. First of all, however, he had to secure a site. Instead of choosing one on the low ground near his palace, which, no doubt, he could have easily done, he selected one on what had become by his time the high road going south from London. Looking back on the controversies of the past thirty years, we might wish he had built on the former, but he was wise to take a drier situation, placing his hospital and, later, his school at the junction of the high road, now called North End, and the " lane that leadeth unto Edgecombe." This has become George Street, from which diverges Park Lane, the " lane that leadeth unto the Park," now covered with residences, but where the old keeper's house still stands. " Edgecombe " has become Addiscombe, historically associated with the great East India Company, who had a military college there.

Whitgift acquired for his site an old inn which he calls the *Checker*,[1] a place known as " Stay cross " (probably a corruption of " Stake cross," from the post on which was marked one of the crosses determining the boundaries of the Archbishop's demesne) and another tenement. These properties were copy-holds, and we know what Whitgift paid for them. Replying to the accusation that he enriched himself out of his office, he gives the several sums, which amounted to £310. While on the subject of cost, it may be stated that the total of building hospital, school-house, and school-master's house came to £2,716, and that the lands and tenements he bought for endowment cost him £2,279, making a grand total of £5,305, which, if multiplied

---

[1] The " Checker " is again mentioned in the accounts of the hospital, and then disappears from history, though it figures in the author's historical romance, *The Arkwrights*, but another road-side inn, the " Swan," long remained and appears in Pyne's water-colour of 1795, kept at the hospital, and seen in Fig. 16, and its old sign is suspended in the audience chamber there.

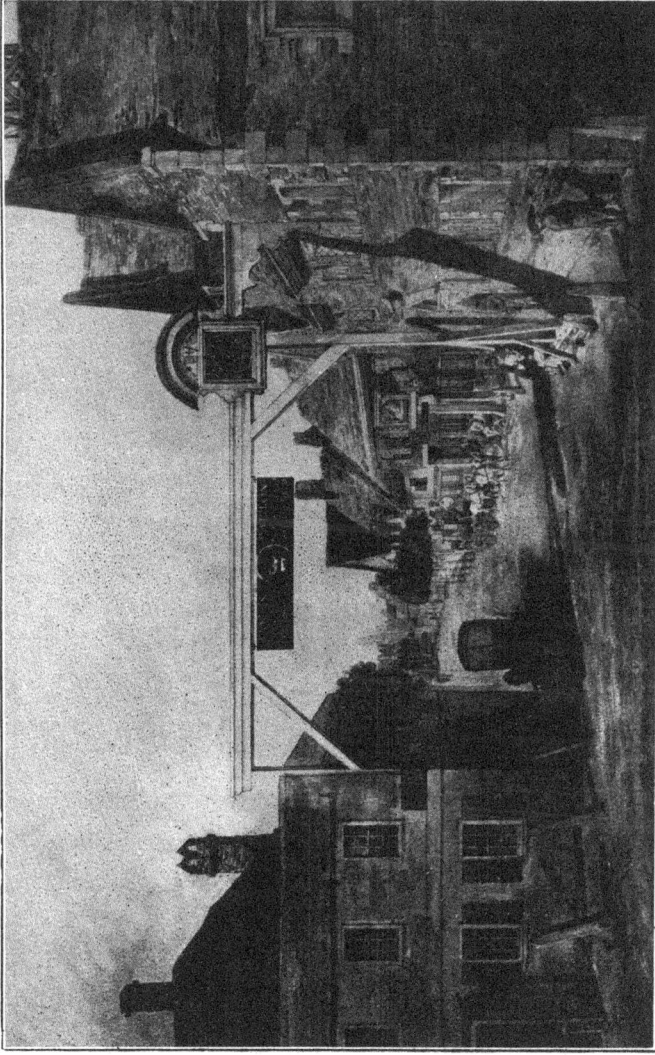

Fig. 16.—WHITGIFT'S HOSPITAL IN 1795
By permission of Messrs H. R. Grubb, Croydon

[Face p. 94

by eight as the relative purchasing power of money in
" pre-war " time, comes to the considerable value of
£42,000.

Personalities.—It will be interesting to linger a while
over these names which appear on early documents.
George Whitgift was a natural son of old Henry Whitgift, of Great Grimsby. His half-brother John left
him by his will the rooms at the hospital which he had
reserved for his own use, and after George's decease
they were to be the lodgings of the Wardens in per-
petuity. Dying in 1611, George Whitgift was buried
in the Church of Holy Faith beneath old St. Paul's,
where his gravestone may be seen to this day. Phillip
Jenkins was a phantom or " figure-head " Warden,
for his name is not attached to any official document,
except, perhaps, on one of the counter-parts of the
deed of gift. " Richard London " was Bancroft,
Whitgift's immediate successor, who founded the
Library at Lambeth Palace. Edward Barker was a
considerable benefactor, and we shall meet him again.
Sir George Paule was the Archbishop's biographer.
Abraham Hartwell was his secretary, M.A., connected
with Trinity College, Cambridge, where Whitgift, who
gave him the Rectory of Toddington, in Bedfordshire,
probably met him. He was a literary man of some note,
translating from the Italian, and spoken of as " an
early evolutionary philosopher."
He was also a member, the last to be admitted, of the
old Society of Antiquaries, before whom he read two
papers. He was about 46 at this time, and we shall
meet his name again in the records. Mathy (Matthew)

Bradburie appears to have married Jane, daughter of one of Whitgift's nieces. Mrs. Sara Copehart, living in the United States, claims descent from that lady. She is keenly interested in everything connected with John Whitgift, and corresponded with the late warden, Alfred Jones, B.A., and the present writer. Michael Murgatrod, in the Archbishop's employ, must have been a man of some importance, for his conspicuous monument was in the parish church before the fire of 1867, and is figured in colours in Corbet Anderson's book on that church. Edward Aylworth was also a benefactor, as we shall see later. He is designated in one place as " armiger," or squire, and generally as of the Middle Temple, whence we infer a lawyer, but also of Hackington, in Kent. His name repeatedly occurs in Whitgift's deeds, acting under his power of attorney. W. Barlow was Whitgift's chaplain, was present at the consecration of the chapel, and afterwards Bishop of Rochester. Francis Butler was descended on his mother's side from the Herons of Edgecombe or Addiscombe, who held land there. He lived long in Croydon, and died 1648 after a life-time spent prominently in local affairs. The Butlers' property came later into the possession of William Draper, son-in-law of John Evelyn, the diarist. Draper rebuilt the house in 1702–3, and Evelyn, who frequently speaks of it in his diary, thought it " one of the best gentlemen's houses in Surrey." In 1809, Addiscombe was sold to the East India Company, who, as we have seen, established a military college there. On dissolution of that Company after the Indian Mutiny, the estate was cut up and covered with streets and houses, the former com-

memorating the names of Anglo-Indian celebrities.[1]
We thus see an unbroken series of links with the present
day.

The story of the Hospital's building, from foundations
to completion, contained in the letters from Samuel
Fynche, Vicar of Croydon, to Whitgift's steward,
Wormeall, and to Whitgift himself, can be seen in the
MSS., Vol. No. 275, at Lambeth Palace Library, and
printed in full in Ducarel's book.   Whitgift was grow-
ing infirm, and apparently left much of his ecclesiastical duties to Bancroft.   This may account for the
superintendence of the building operations being left
to Fynche, who gave faithful solicitude to them.   So
interesting a light do these letters throw upon the
methods of the work that some extracts are here given.

" From Croydon, this Friday, the VIIIth of Februarie,
Anno 1596.   To the moste reverende Father in God my
verie good Lorde the Archbishop of Canterburie, his
grace at Lambeth, with all speed. . . .   Wolmer was
here to view your worke.   And he sayeth that he
cannot be here himself : but he will appoint one from
Westminster to be here, who will not come under
xviij*d* the day, and his laborer xijd.   Hilarie sayeth
he canne bring one presently whome he knoweth, and
will warrant to take the charge and discharge it with
credit, for xvjd a day ;   and laborers we can have
enow : thers vli. [£5] a yeare, saved in ij*d* a day wages,[2]
and beside the master workeman must be here still
[continuously] to conferre with the carpenter. . .   The
yarde ys all defenced in, strong and saffe.   This day

---

[1] Corbet Andersons' *Chronicle of Croydon* and notes given to the present
writer by Mr. Clarence G. Paget, of Croydon.
[2] A little out in his arithmetic !

we made an ende in pulling down as yet. Nowe we take mortar-makinge in hand, clensing and levellinge the grounde; and by Monday come sevennighte, Hilarie saith, we shall be readye for the foundacon and bricklayer. Weeks the bricklayer hath been at your brick-clamps, and he commendes them for very good. We have our sande from Dubbers [Duppas] Hill: for the parke fayleth.

Samuel Fynche, Vycar."

" Blease hath begune the grounde worke nexte the highway leadinge to London; and finding that grounde made and false, digged the trench alonge the door unto some iiii foote deepe, and iii foote wide . . . and findinge firme grounde, they have filled up that trenche with greate flinte and small stone, and brickbatts and rubbishe not confusedly, but orderlye layed in, and rammed stronglye, course upon course, strong and sure. . . . Four loads of flinte, which come to x*s*, will save one thousand of bricks at xvi*s*. . . . The bearer hereof ys Wm. Tagburne, who had vli [£5] of me this morning to bye two horses tomorrow in Smithfeilde. . . . The laborers have digged up iiii skulls and the bones of deade persons in the trench that they are nowe in digginge, next the highway leadinge to the Parke.[1] I thank God, our groundworke is greatlye commended of all that view the same. And I hope well that will like his Grace at his cominge; for yt is not slubbered uppe, but strongely done.

Sa. Fynche."—To Wormeall.

---

[1] It has been supposed that these bones represent an engagement that took place in 1264 between the forces of Henry III. and the Londoners after the battle of Lewes.

He encloses a copy of the first bond or contract mentioned in this connection, namely, to supply the free-stone for the doorways and windows, and to work and set up the same. The price was to be 9d. the foot for the windows and 10d. the foot for the doors.

In Letter V Fynche unburdens his soul to Wormeall about Blease, the bricklayer, who had been taking too much upon himself. He gets a sound rating from the reverend clerk of the works, for he seems to have been doing a little trickery on his own account by making men who came on the job pay him 2d. a day as a sort of commission and condition of not being pushed on.

Letter VI refers with dissatisfaction to the bricks made by one Rednap and stacked in park and yard :—
" Fain would he have excused himselfe, but his handie work spoke against him, and we were so round with him, that he burste into tears, saying, he was never the like served in anie worke ; he was ashamed of it, he could not excuse it, yt was the wickedness and deceitfulnesse of the yearthe."

Fynche sends a plan from the " freemasons " relative to the outer gate, and receives from Lambeth instructions as follows :—

" The Armes over the doore must be without helmet and mantelling ; and must be the arms of the See of Canterbury, viz., the Pall [pallium] in pale with the nowe Archbishop's armes, and the yeare of the Lord under them, viz., 1597. Over the said armes a free-stone square, with theis words in great letters, viz., SANCTAE TRINITATI SACR. On the bare places over the gate, this sentence following to be written in great capital letters, *viz.* :—Pro. 28. QUI DAT PAUPERI NON INDEGEBIT."

The hospital took nearly four years to build, having been begun, as we have seen, on January 17th, 1596, and finished by September 29th, 1599. The School buildings were not completed till three years later. The present writer has made enquiries, but no contemporary drawings of the hospital exist. There are, however, three sources from which we can draw a mental picture of it, when new from the builder's hands. Stow (*c.* 1525–1605) speaks of it in his *Survey of London*, 1598, as " a fair brick building builded like a college," that is, round a quadrangle. Ducarel's plate, dated 1755, a hundred and fifty-six years later, indicates a classical form of gateway with a round arch and Corinthian-like pilasters. Although the appearance of ashler (worked stones) in the general front may be ignored as due to the slurring of architectural details common at this period, we may take it that the draughtsman has been at some pains to portray the actual form of the gateway. Pyne's water-colour, besides vividly restoring for us the life in Croydon of his day with the " Swan," the coaches and chaises, the old pensioners watching the " busy " scene and the wigged gentleman, indicates a detail of some importance, to wit, stonework in the windows. This is the more significant in that some have suggested that the windows were of moulded brick, after the single example of such in the kitchen, ignoring Fynche's letter quoted on p. 99.

The Hospital Chapel, a very simple descendant of the

PLATE X.

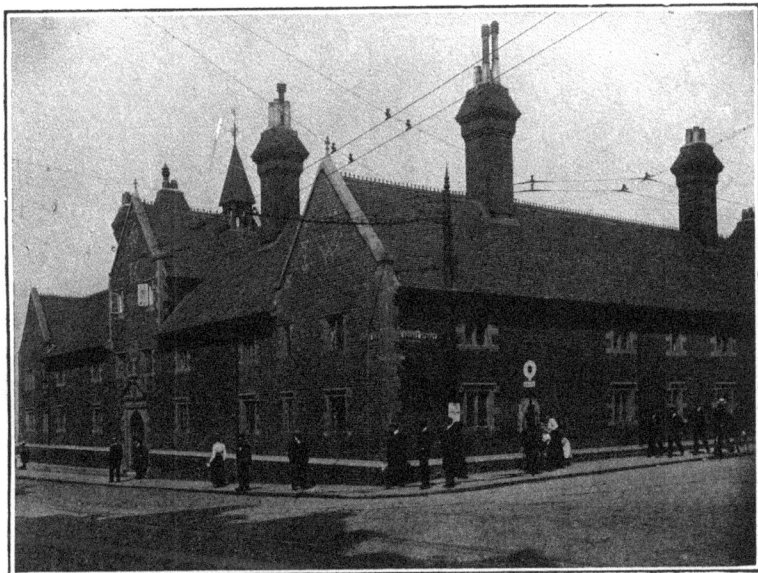

Fig. 17.—WHITGIFT'S HOSPITAL, PRESENT DAY
By permission of Messrs H. R. Grubb, Croydon

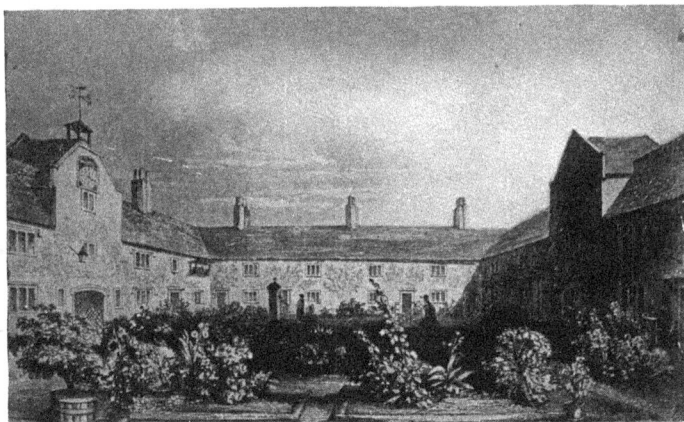

Fig. 18.—QUADRANGLE IN 1840
By permission of Messrs H. R. Grubb, Croydon

[*Face p.* 100

ancient and beautiful edifices, was consecrated by
Bishop Bancroft on Monday, July 9th, 1599, and by
the Michaelmas of that year the real life of Whitgift's
Hospital began, that date remaining for long after the
commencement of its official year.

Before we enter his hospital to explore it and afterwards follow its internal history, it will be well to glance
at the INFLUENCES which led Whitgift to give it its
form and constitution.   He must have been well aware
of the ancient custom of building hospitals, and, in his
younger days, have witnessed the widespread misery
created by their extensive dissolution.   There were
several existing hospitals surviving that Dissolution,
notably Ewelme in Oxfordshire, from which to choose,
and from which to leave out elements in his plans.
He would not dedicate his house to any saint, believing,
like his successor Abbot, that such should be given to
God alone.   He therefore dedicates to the Holy Trinity,
a name ever since attaching to his hospital.   He would
not, of course, have his pensioners pray for his soul,
but they were to give daily thanks for their founder.
There was to be a resident head, whom he calls Warden,
not Master, later to be chosen by the inmates from
among themselves.   They were a corporation, with full
ownership of large landed endowments and an ample
home with inner and outer gate-house and gardens,
bowling green, orchard, and even forest trees were
planted.   They were to be there, in his thought, "for
ever," and his successors in office were to be their
patrons and protectors.   How far Whitgift's ideals were
realised, subsequent history will tell us.

General View.—The Hospital of the Holy Trinity

H

stands at the junction of the North End and George Street, giving the normal alignment to each. On the three gables, letters in blue brick indicate alternately by J.W., J.C., and J.W. again, John Whitgift and Joannes Cantuariensis. While the schoolmaster's house stood, it also had J.W. on its front.

Entering by what is now a mean portal, one is impressed by the wonderful transition from turmoil without to perfect peace within. But what strikes the observant visitor more is the marked fitness of things. Ranged along the four sides of an ample quadrangle are the two-storied cottage-homes, dominated only by the simple outer and inner gate-houses. Above the archway of the latter are Whitgift's (now the Warden's) sitting-room and bedroom. (See Fig. 19.) The door and two latticed windows to the left are those of the hall, the windows above of the audience chamber. Aloft is the one remaining original chimney-stack, with four separate flues. In the corner is the entrance to the old kitchen ; thence all round to the outer gate-house are the brothers' and sisters' single rooms, warm and sufficiently lighted. Over the arch of the outer gate-house is the window of the muniment room —Whitgift's " house of evidences "—and the one-handed clock face. The little pent-houses are modern, but quite fitting additions. (Cf. Lyford, Fig. 11.) Following these round we come to the entrance—alas ! an ill-adapted modern annex—to the little chapel, apparently " tucked away " into a corner. It occupies, however, the gable-end of the south side and, when further examined, will be found, though by no means ornate, perfectly adapted to the intention of its founder.

PLATE XI.

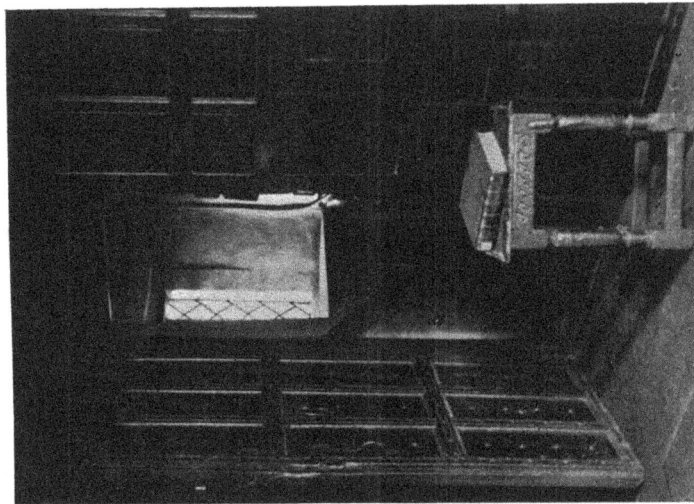

Fig. 20.—STRONG DOOR AND JOINT STOOL.

[Face p. 102

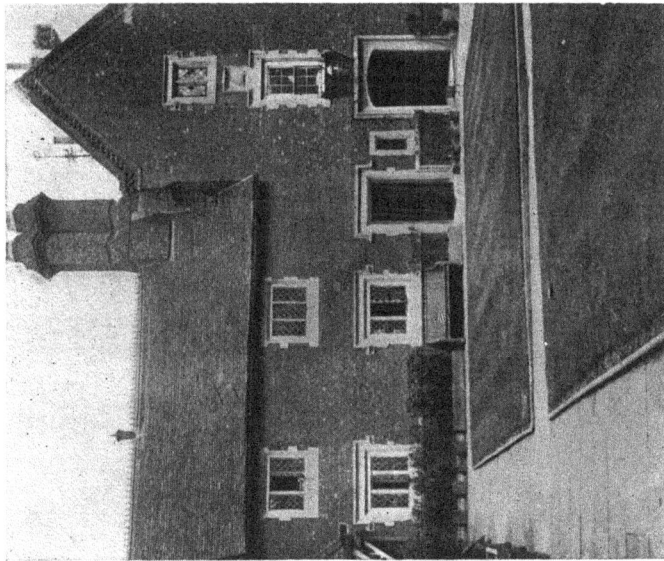

Fig. 19.—WARDEN'S QUARTERS AND HALL

There are ornamental blue bricks above the window externally, and a tablet bearing the inscription—

EBORACENSIS

HANC FENESTRA[M])

FIERI FECIT

1597

The modest citizen of York who caused this window to be made was William Thornhill, Whitgift's chaplain, and we shall see later what the window cost him. Speaking of it, about 20 years ago, Mr. Colerick Smith, architect, said that here was Gothic work executed by a man with classical ideas. The rough-hewn benches within have no backs to encourage slumbering, and very simple poppy-heads. Upon the west wall is a contemporary portrait of Whitgift in a carved frame of the period with a Latin inscription, not revealing a very forgiving spirit, of which the following is a translation.

Above : I have done what I could. I was able to do what was given by Christ. [Do] better if thou canst, Ill-will.

Below : Behold a true portrait of that Principal who first built this dwelling to the Holy Three.

If Whitgift had his Puritan opponents in mind, he might have remembered that they were mostly poor men.

The archways have the depressed four-centred character of the Elizabethan period, and the wooden window-frames will be found to have the ovalo and fillet mould-ing prevailing throughout the entire building. Passing under the arch of the inner gate-house, we find a

typically moulded oaken doorway and a short flight of
steps, at the top of which is the strong door opening on
to the **Audience Chamber.** This unpretentious room
forms part of the quarters which Whitgift reserved to
himself, is 25 feet long by 15 feet wide, and is partly
open to the roof, which is only ceiled at the height of
nearly 13 feet. It is wainscoted throughout up to
$7\frac{1}{2}$ feet with small panels enclosed in unmitred framing,
and is characteristic of the period. The chief ornament
of this room is the overmantel (Fig. 21). It is boldly
carved in Renaissance style, though the Tudor element
lingers in the roses. A short alley-way leads to the
private room in the gate-house closed by a door, the
exact counterpart of that at the summit of the stair, to
wit, " two-ply," nine-panelled, bolted through and with
characteristic furniture. This room is wainscoted
like the Audience chamber, but to a little greater height.
A door in the wainscot, with beautiful hinges, opens on
to a little winding stair lighted by a tiny dormer. This
leads up to the **sleeping chamber,** which is a replica in
miniature of the audience room. An extraordinary
feature of the strong door which closes this room con-
sists in additions to the usual lock. Two iron bars sink
into the wall when the door is closed, evidently to
prevent the hinges being forced, while two apparent
bolt-heads unscrew and at the bottom are bolts turned
by a special key. It has been assumed that this was a
provision against violence to Whitgift, who suffered
from the enmity, or at least " mislike," of some of his
contemporaries. Were this so, and the special locks
could only be worked from the outside, Whitgift would
have to depend upon his personal servant to release

PLATE XII.

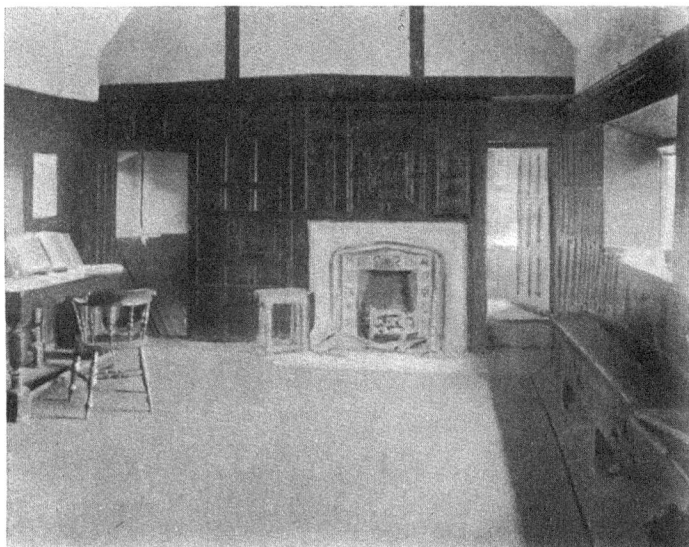

Fig. 21.—AUDIENCE CHAMBER

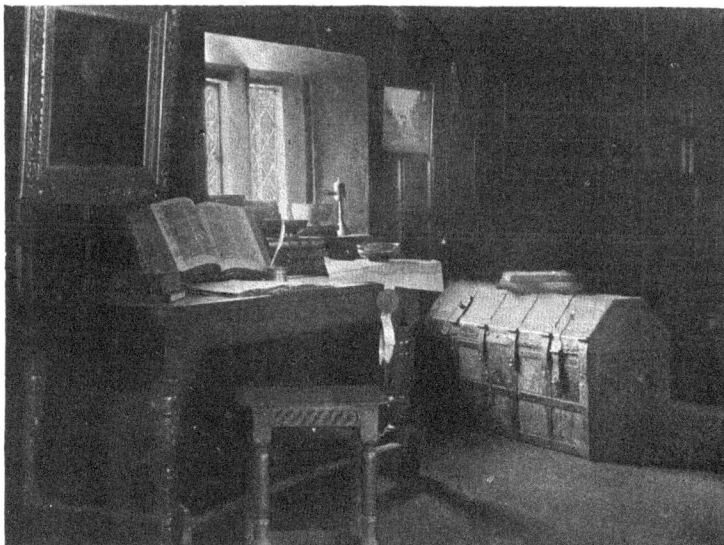

Fig. 22.—A CORNER IN AUDIENCE CHAMBER WITH
TREASURE CHEST

[*Face p. 104*

him of a morning.   But it is not to be supposed that
he often used this chamber, and it seems more likely
that he had a particular reason for preventing this
room being entered *in his absence,* and that he kept
the special key himself.   At the opposite end of the
audience chamber, a few steps lead up to the kitchen,
and a door, now fastened up, opened into a room in the
north wing, where, probably, Whitgift's servant slept.

The Hall is immediately beneath the Audience
chamber, and corresponds with it in area, while its
ceiling is crossed by intersecting joists.   It was served,
at its northern end, directly from the kitchen, through
a buttery-hatch.   Its casement windows open upon the
quadrangle and rear-court respectively, and some of
them retain their original stained glass.   Of this we
may note, in a west window, a crown with Whitgift's
motto—*Vincit qui patitur*—and the border round his
arms, while on the east side are the complete arms of
Edward Aylworth, whose name we have already seen
and shall meet again.   The fireplace is of Elizabethan-
Jacobean type.   **The Kitchen,** now used as a wash-
house, retains its wide open fireplace, its dresser within
the thickness of the party-wall, the buttery-hatch
opening from it into the hall, some old dishes and
chargers, and a little recess for the reserve of dough
against the next batch of baking.

Original Warden's Quarters.—Writers on New College, Oxford, founded by Bishop Wykeham in 1379,
speak of the Warden having his *traditional* chambers[1]
over the outer gate-house, and it is reasonable to think
that the Wardens at Croydon had their quarters there

[1] *Discovery,* Oct., 1924.

during the lives of John and George Whitgift. By the side of the room now used as the clerk's office, next to the outer gate-house, a winding stair leads to a solitary strong door like those in the Audience chamber. This opens into a room, now the living-room of the clock-keeper, which, in turn, gave access to the muniment-room immediately over the gate by another strong door. From the first room a stair still leads to an upper floor, partly used as the sleeping apartment of the clock-keeper, partly for the clock. But the clock was origin-ally not in the gate-house, being as late as Pyne's picture of 1795 close to the south-west gable. Who, then, should have occupied these rooms but the Warden *before* he had been " translated " to the inner gate-house ? It has been found that the chimney of the muniment room had been blocked by a slab of stone— perhaps an after-thought to prevent burglars from descending by way of the flue ! Many years ago now, Mr. John Jones, the secretary, found, amongst a bundle of keys, one which would turn the lock of that long-closed door of the long disused and forgotten muniment room, and entered. He found it canopied in cobwebs and carpeted with dust. Here was a table with a raised rim for counting the " wages " of the members, and, far more important, a great chest stuffed full with a confused mass of documents, leather-covered little deed-boxes, and, in the midst, two priceless mazers. The late Mr. Frewer, one of the governors, spent two years in sorting and tabulating the documents. The frame of the door had been plastered over on the outside, and the woodwork looks as fresh as if it had been fixed yesterday. In re-adjustment after Mr. Jones' discovery, the frame and door were reversed. The inventory quoted in the next chapter, p. 129, mentions the contents of the muniment room, and bears the date 1634. It is evident, therefore, that the door was last closed and the room forgotten some time, perhaps soon, after this. There is no later inventory extant.

CHAPTER XII

WHITGIFT'S HOSPITAL—*continued*

The Bell.—It is fitting that this chapter should open with the tolling of a bell, for its bell is far and away the oldest thing in the Hospital, where it has, throughout three centuries and more, struck the passing hours. For facts concerning the clock and its bell the writer is entirely indebted to what was written by his dear old friend, Alfred Jones, late warden, and published by him in the *Reliquary* under title " The Romance of our Hospital Bell." In 1608 a change of bells took place at Lincoln Cathedral, some smaller being replaced by " Great Tom." In 1610 these entries occur in the ledger book. "Master John Shaw, clerk to the Chamber of London, gave unto Trinity Hospital a clock and diall." A little lower down—" The foresayed Master Shaw gave a bell unto our Hospital, and payed for enlarging and making stronger the Clock House—3l." [£3]. Some years ago, the bell-cote underwent repairs, and Alfred Jones had an opportunity of examining the bell. After giving the dimensions—it is only about a foot and a half high—he transcribes the inscriptions. Round the shoulder runs—OREMUS PRO BONO STATU DECANI ET CAPITULI ECCLESIÆ CATHEDRALIS BEATÆ MARIÆ DE LINCOLNÆ ; Let us pray for the good estate of Dean and Chapter of the Cathedral Church of the Blessed Mary of Lincoln. Along the rim, the lettering

is—DALYSON MILES FIRMARIUS HUIUS MANERII DE
GRETWEL ME FIERI FECIT QUARTO APRILIS ANNO DMI
1414. The hardest part to decipher then, after three
centuries of striking from the *outside*, was the year.
Jones says—" The years 1511 and 1596 have been previously suggested. There is, however, no visible mark
of a curved numeral. Relics of the figures are all
straight lines, which, carefully completed, give the
result in the text."

If we accept the author's rendering of the lower
inscription, it reads in English—Dalyson, knight and
farmer [occupier] of this manor of Gretwel, caused me
to be made the fourth of April the year of our Lord
1414. Gretwel, now Greetwell, is a small parish two
miles from Lincoln. Much to his regret, the present
writer missed an opportunity of photographing the
bell, but Mr. Maurice Houghton photographed it when
rehung, and his print can be seen in the Croydon Public
Library.

Mazers.—The next oldest treasure belonging to the
hospital is the " senior " mazer-bowl (see Fig. 24). It
bears the London hall-mark 1508-9. The later and
larger mazer is silver-gilt throughout, and has the
London hall-mark of 1599-1600. Common sense leads
us to remotest pre-history for the origin of a drinking-
cup or any bowl for holding liquids where a shell would
not suffice. In warmer latitudes than our own, a
gourd, cut through and dried, was a calabash (Arabic,
qar, a gourd, and *aibas*, dry), an excellent drinking-cup
which could be left as a " tumbler," or made to stand
by a little scraping or cutting of the under side, have a
lid of the other half and be decorated according to

fancy. In mediæval times, when something more ornate than the simple beech-wood bowl, turned on the lathe, was demanded, the *spotted* maple was employed, a short foot of silver or silver-gilt was added, as well as a decorated or inscribed rim and a central boss or " print."[1] These features occur in the older mazer, all of precious metal. These mazers (German, *maser*, a spot) were in use amongst persons of high degree from the thirteenth to the sixteenth century, after which " standing cups " and other more artistic designs superseded them. For lesser folk, plainer devices sufficed, and of these three have remained to the hospital; they are of beech-wood, painted, and have the following legends around them : **Comfort the comfortless Forget not thy beginning, think of thine end. What sirrah hold thy peace, thirst satisfied cease.** Though mazers are mentioned in inventories as early as the thirteenth century, none of that time are now known as extant. Two preserved at Harbledown Hospital are of the fourteenth century, one of them being of Edward II.'s reign and the oldest in England. The Brackenbridge mazer of 1534 is figured in the article *Plate* in the *Encyclopædia Britannica,* and was sold in 1908 for £2,300. The rim-band extends quite one-third down and is inscribed in Lombardic characters. The smaller mazer, the " bowl tipt with silver and gilt," mentioned later in the hospital inventories, is not so large as the Brackenbridge mazer, but is quite as artistic. The print is elaborately and beautifully engraved. The larger one, Dean Neville's mazer,

[1] It has been suggested that the print represents the core of a gourd from which the fibres for nourishing the seeds radiate : if so, it is an interesting survival of a very ancient custom.

PLATE XIII.

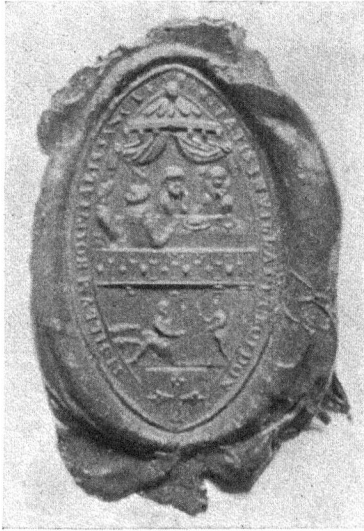

Fig. 23.—CORPORATE SEAL

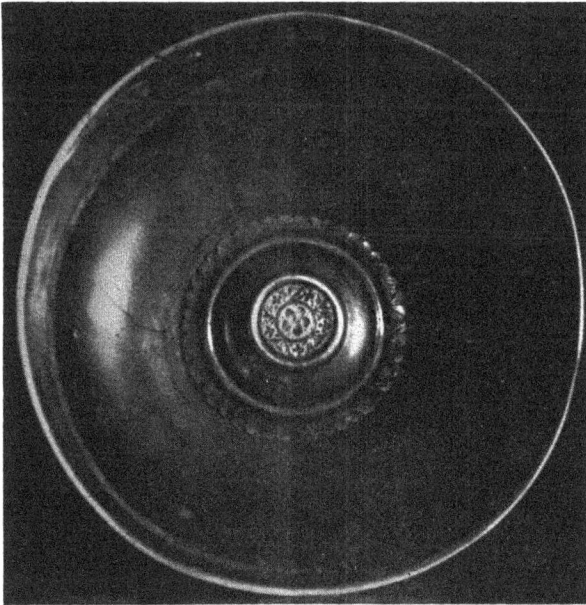

Fig. 24.—OLDEST MAZAR

is entirely of metal, and has underneath a coat of arms which are apparently the donor's.[1]

The humbler drinking-cups, though obviously far less precious than the mazers, are rare, because, wanting metal protection, they were the more easily destroyed. All are now in the South Kensington Museum. But mention is made of them in the Ledger books, to the investigation of which we will presently turn.

Free School and Schoolmasters.—It would be tedious to quote at any length from Whitgift's 21 statutes, but a few references are necessary, the better to understand the management and history of the hospital. No mention of school or schoolmaster occurs in the charter of incorporation, and the attachment of a free school was evidently an after-thought, though there were abundant precedents at the time. Although the words "brethren" and "sisters" do not occur in the charter, the schoolmaster, according to the statutes, was to be a poor brother and "a parson well qualified for that function, that is to saye, an honest man, learnede in the Greeke and Latin tongues, and able to write well, if possible it may be, whiche poore brother appointed to that office . . . shall have for his lodginge and dwellinge place . . . that howse which I have builded for that purpose, adjoining to the saide Hospitall, and nere unto the saide schoolehouse, together with suche backsides and grounds as I have appointed to be annexed to the said

---

[1] This Dean Neville, Thomas Nevile of the endorsement, "Mr. Dr. Nevell" of the benefactions, was Dean of Canterbury, "overseer" of Whitgift's will, Master of Magdalen College, Oxford, and Chaplain, both to Queen Elizabeth and to Whitgift. He was a scion of the ancient and once powerful house of that name. The arms at the base of the mazer are much quartered, but include the Neville cross saltire and some of the differences.

howse . . . and shall also have the some of twentye pounds yearely for his stipande . . . together with other further comodities of corne or wood as hereafter shal happen to be allotted to other of the poore brethren of the saide Hospitall." His appointment was in the hands of the Archbishop.

Although the word " parson " does not necessarily imply that the schoolmaster was to be a cleric, in practice he was such, and far too much power was placed in his hands by Whitgift, who clearly was not a business man. The schoolmaster had not only to be recorder, accountant, and joint claviger, or key-keeper, but had as well a share in the handling of money. On the other hand, the Warden, also a poor brother, but not required to be learned, in fact, too often unable to sign his name, was to be elected by a majority vote at a meeting of the schoolmaster and other brethren, the former having a casting vote. The annals of the hospital show how unwise were these arrangements. The moral status of the lower clergy at this time and for long afterwards was none too high, and the further history of the hospital reveals not only mismanagement and neglect, but more than one instance of irregularity, not to say flagrant dishonesty, on the part of a schoolmaster.

Records.—There were to be three Ledger books for various specified entries, but in practice but one at a time seems to have been used by the clerical scribe and accountant. From these books, kept under the care of the wardens, Alfred Jones compiled a valuable work on the domestic life of the hospital. Unfortunately, this book has never been published. From some extracts, however, from the Ledger books, made by the present writer, and many by Alfred Jones, he is able to give several interesting illustrations.

Benefactions.—The first page of Fynche's entry in the Ledger book (he was practically *fac totum* during his lifetime) is here transcribed, *verbatim et literatim*, except money statements. " Mr. Wyllm Myll Esquyre, was at the Charge of the fforce [pump] for Lead, Soader [Solder], Brassworke and Workmanship, whiche coste hym—£48, 16s, 11d.[1] Mr. Wyllm Thornehill his Gr. Chapelane, was at the Charge of ye greate Wyndoe in the Chapple for stone, Yron and glasse Worke, whiche coste hym—£12, 16s, 8d.

Mr. Edwarde Aylworth gent. was at the charge of the Casements & Glazinge of the Hawle & yt cost hym—£3, 4s, 2d.[2]

Mr. John Bond gent. was at the charge, for the Casements & Glazinge of the Scholehouse, & yt coste hym—£6, 13s, 10d.

Mr. Hartwell his Gr. servaunte, bestowed the gyfte of the Byble in the Chapple.

Mr. Wormeall his Gr. servaunte, bestowed the gyfte of the X Commandments in the Chapple.

Mr. Parker gent. gave the standinge Cuppe that ys plated aboute Wth Sylver. *See Inventory, but since lost.*

Mr. Webbe, his Gr. Chapelaine, bestowed the gyfte

---

[1] This heavy charge, for that time, probably included the sinking of the well. The list of benefactions goes on till 1640. In 1635–6 the pump was renewed and £15 12s. made by selling the old metal. In the petition against taking Wandle water in 1610, much was made of the cost to Sir Francis Carew in setting up a " force " at Beddington.

[2] A later insertion reads, " and he gave at his death xxvj rugg gownes " ; these were probably of fustian. By his will, Aylworth gave 20 similar gowns to Abbot's Hospital. See next chapter. Indeed, so many were the benefactions in kind, as well as money, that much expense was saved to the foundation.

of all those trees wherewth the Orcharde ys Planted.

Mr. Doctor Nevell, dean of Canterbury, bestowed the gyfte of a Cuppe of Sylver & double gylte, Weyghinge xxix ounces.

Mr. Barker, register of ye highe comission, gave twentie nobles a year for ever to ye Hospital and Dame Susan, his wife, gave fortie in monie to purchase Land, two worthy benefactors."

This is the Edwarde Barker whose name we have seen in the endorsements and who, by a deed exhibited in the audience chamber, with his wife gave a rent-charge of £6 13s. 4d. per annum for 1,000 years upon the site of Lancaster College in St. Paul's Church Yard. The deed is so worded that the present occupiers, Messrs. Cook, still pay the Hospital the fixed sum of £6 13s. 4d a year. This document is further interesting for the series of family coats of arms with which it is decorated, one being the shield of Lucy, displaying three pikes or luces, the bearings of that Justice Shallow, pilloried in Shakespeare's *Merry Wives of Windsor*; and also for the two central seals being attached through a gold angel.

The story goes that once, in his earlier days, Shakespeare got into trouble with Sir Thomas Lucy, a Warwickshire magnate of old family, for poaching. Reference to the Lucy arms on the Barker deed will help readers to appreciate the sharpest point in the satire. " The *pike* is the *luce* of heraldry. . . . There is no earlier example borne in English heraldry than is afforded by the pikes on the arms of the family of Lucy." Moule (heraldry of Fish), quoted in *Imperial Dictionary*.

Slender: " All his successors, gone before him, hath done it ; and all his ancestors, that come after him, may : [write *Armigero*] they may give the dozen white luces in their coat."

Shallow : " It is an old coat."

Sir Hugh Evans (a Welsh parson) : " The dozen white *louses* do become an old coat ; it agrees well, passant ; it is a familiar beast to man, and signifies love."

Hartwell's Bible is a folio edition of 1575, in black letter, popularly styled the " Treacle Bible," from the word *balm* or *balsam* being rendered *triacle* in two places in the text as well as in Cranmer's preface. This was a good translation at the time when treacle or molasses, as we understand the terms, were unknown, but then meant a viscid curative substance, such as Venice treacle.[1] The Old Testament portion still remains in the Audience chamber.

Register of Admissions and Deaths.—The beautiful penmanship of Samuel Fynche is here seen, clear as if written yesterday, on some of the first pages of the first Ledger book. In the opening lines we meet again with Thomas Elton, of the first twelve, as well as at the election to be quoted presently, though here spelt with an *h*. Whitgift clearly relaxed his own statute that a man might not lodge his wife, out of compassion for this old man's blindness, and the rule, once broken, seems to have made the way open for men to bring their wives in with them. Elton had a double allowance

---

[1] The once famous Venice treacle had a multitude of ingredients which might well have included portions from snakes, for Cranmer, in his preface, says, " Out of the most venomous worms [serpents] is made treacle, the most sovereign medicine for the preservation of man's health in time of danger."

(2s. a week), while Whitgift lived. Harrie Jefferies is probably the Henry Geoffrey of the charter, and so is, we may be sure, Robert Curtis of the letters patent. Widow Alice Dibble may have been the wife of Richard Dibble, whose name has disappeared. Seeing she was 88 years old when admitted, it is not surprising that her name heads the list of deaths next year. It is remarkable and significant that Fynche writes " Prior," a term not used by Whitgift, instead of " Schoolmaster."

There is a touch of pathos clinging to these initial entries, which are here transcribed from the first pages of each series, *verbatim et literatim* :—

" THE ADMITTANCE and Entraunce of the Warden, Prior & pore Brethren & systers into the Hospitall of the Holy Trynitie.

Thomas Elthon of the parish of Croydon, Blynde & of the Age of lxxj years : entred wth his aged wyfe, the seconde day of October.   Anno D$\overline{m}$ 1599.

Roberte Fynge, of the sayd parishe, Sole, & of the Age of lxxiiij years : Entred the said sayd [*sic*] seconde day of October, Anno D$\overline{m}$ 1599.

Alice Dyble of the sayd parishe, Wydoe, and of the Age of lxxxviij years : Entred the thirde day of the said October.   Anno p'd$\overline{co}$.

Elsabeth Otes, of the said parish, Widoe, and of the Age of lxiiij years : Entred the vth day of October above said.   Anno p'd$\overline{co}$ [aforesaid].

Harrie Jefferie, of the said parish, Sole, and of the Age of lxxxx years : Entred the xijth day of October, as before.

Roberte Curtis, of the sayd Parishe, sometyme his Gr. pore servaunt, of the Age of lij years.   Admitted but not yet entred. [His *youth*! the age limit being reduced for Archbishop's servants.]

Anne Saltemarshe, of the said parishe, Widoe, & of the Age of lxxiiij. Admitted the xjth of Januarie & entred the xvijth of marche, Anno p'dco.

Ambrose Brygges, mr. of Arts, & qualified according to his Gr. Constitutions, in that case provided ; married, & of the Age of xlviij years, entred Scholemaister the xxxjth Day of Marche, Anno Dm. 1600." (Here there was no age limit.)

" THE DEATHS or REMOVINGS of Warden, Prior & the pore of the Hospitall of the Holye Trinitye.

Alyce Dyble, Widoe, Deceassed the xvijth day of November Anno Dm 1600.

. . . .

Ambrose Brygs, Scholemaister, Departed the xxiiijth day of June 1601.

Roberte Curtys Deceassed the vth Day of Januarii, 1601.

Harrye Jeffrey Deceassed the xxviijth Day of Aprill, 1603.

Roberte Fynge deceassed the ixth Day of Auguste Anno Dm 1603.

Our Moste Gratious Lorde John Whitgifte, Doctor of Dyvynitie, Archbushop of Canterburie, Primate & Metropolitan of all Englande Lorde of the moste Honorable privie Counsell, both to our late Queen Elizabeth, as also to our Dreade soveraigne Kynge James, that nowe ys : Founder of the famous Hospitall of the Holye Trinitie in Croydon : Deceased at Lambeth the xxixth Day of Februarii & was buried in the Chapple of Croydon, where his pore people are placed [S. choir aisle]

I

the seconde Day of Marche followinge.   And his funerall
rytes were solemnized the xxviith Day of the same
moneth Anno D̄m 1604, Anno D̄m Regni nri [nostri]
Regis Jacobi secondi.

Father Outred deceassed the xxjth Day of June,
    1604.
Christofer Fennar resygned & gave over his place
    the vth day of Juely Anno Dm 1604."

All the events registered at this period are dated in
the "old style" according to which those which
happened between Jan. 1st and March 25th were
reckoned as in the previous year.   In placing them
according to the new style, inaugurated in 1752, we
have to put forward the year three months and add
eleven days.
    Thus we have :—

Whitgift's death, Feb. 29, 1603, *old style*, 1604 *new style*
His burial   Mar. 2, 1603   ,,   ,,   1604   ,, ,,
His funeral   Mar. 27, 1604   ,,   ,,   1604   ,, ,,
James' accn.   Mar. 24, 1602   ,,   ,,   1603   ,, ,,

James I. had thus just entered his second year on
the date of Whitgift's funeral, and when he presented
Samuel Fynche, as we shall see presently, he was
already nearly a year on the throne of England.

The Wardens.—Alfred Jones gave the writer the
following notes concerning the wardens :—
    Phillip Jenkins, the "well beloved" of the letters,
was, as we have observed, a phantom warden.   Robert

Foster was admitted as warden on the 2nd of April, 1600, and is mentioned as late Usher of the Archbishop's hall and *first* warden. If not a phantom, he was no more than a " figurehead," for, while he lived, Whitgift kept the administration in his hands, acting through Fynche as governor. Foster died in 1604, was buried, and his funeral sermon preached by Vicar Fynche the next day. Edward Burton was the next warden. Whitgift had now died, and the election of Burton according to the statutes is thus recorded in the Ledger book : " Mr. Edwarde Burton Mr. of Artes, late fellowe of Gonville and Caius College Chambridge, Commissarye of London & officiall to ye Archdeacon of Middlesexe, of the age of three score and twoe yearse was admitted and sworne a brother of this Hospitall xxth day of December Anno Dmn. 1604."

"The Election of ye Warden [written in margin]. The foresayde Mr. Edwarde Burton was elected Warden of this Hospitall xxist day of ye said moneth according to ye statutes wth ye full consente of al ye Brethren then present whose names are hereunder written, viz, John Ireland Schoole Mr., John Holande Francis Beste Anthony Lavebeye Edwarde Smith Thomas Elton John Jenkins Reynalde Scroobie George Newton Nicholas Feilde. This election was made in the presence of Samuell Fynche Governoure Michael Murgatrod George Paule."

An Audit.—There are many more documents at the hospital, but a few more extracts must suffice. William Nicholson, schoolmaster, delivers his audit in the hall on December 4th, 1618, according to statute. After he has shown his figures and balance in somewhat irregular manner, the brethren present sign, some their names quite well, others including the Warden, Robert Jenkins, make their marks, against which Nicholson writes their names.

Edward Burton and Alfred Jones were the only wardens who were men of learning; all the rest during nearly three hundred years were otherwise, yet in all that time there is only one record of a Warden being expelled for dishonesty. Jasper Yardley, appointed Warden in 1621, may be taken as a partial exception, for he resigned to become master of Abbot's Hospital at Guildford, a position implying business capacity. He left a benefaction to Whitgift's, and gave £10 for panelling the chapel.

Subsequent Care by Archbishops.—Notwithstanding Whitgift's pathetic appeal to his successors that they would " in the bowells of Christ " have a fatherly care of his pensioners, this does not seem to have been generally manifested. Between Whitgift's death and 1771 (167 years) there appear to have been only nine visitations, the last, so far as the records show, being the only personal one, that by Archbishop Manners Sutton in 1812, when the accounts of Schoolmaster Dr. John Rose were examined. This eventuated in his being found guilty in court of misappropriating the funds to the amount of over £760. A hundred years earlier, John Cæsar, both Schoolmaster and Vicar of Croydon, had to sign a bond not to take any of his salary of £20 a year till a debt of £184 which he acknowledged to the hospital has been repaid by him.

Schoolmasters.—Ducarel gives a list of these up to 1783, which is date of his book, as follows :—

1600. Ambrose Brydges (*i.e.*, Brygges, who " departed " next year).
1601. John Ireland.
1606. Robert Davies (expelled 1616).
1616. Wm. Nicholson.
1629. John Webb.
1651. Thos. Gray.
1668. Wm. Crow.

1675. John Shepherd.
1681. John Cæsar (defaulter).
1711. Henry Mills.
1742. Samuel Staveley.
John Taylor Lamb.
James Hodgson, " now chaplain " 1783.

Shepherd and Mills were somewhat distinguished men, Mills in particular, and Ducarel writes of them at length. It is possible that Cæsar was a son or grandson of Sir Charles Cæsar, Master of the Rolls in Charles I.'s time, or descended from some other member of this distinguished family of remarkable name. The first in England was Adelmare Cesare, of Italian descent, who was physician to Queens Mary and Elizabeth. His son, Julius Cæsar, was a judge in Elizabeth's time, and of lavish generosity, of whom we saw something in the first chapter, p. 6; another son was Henry, Dean of Ely. If these people were John Cæsar's relations, his preferment and lenient treatment may be explained.[1]

Solemn Admonitions.—This attempt to restore, in some small measure, the social life of long past years, would be deficient were we to pass unnoticed some of these quaint events at Whitgift's Hospital, the more so as the slightly younger sister at Guildford seems to have been happily free of them. Jones laboriously copied out most, if not all, of these in their original orthography. Two admonitions will be found in the next

[1] *Dict. National Biography.*

chapter because they bear on Archbishop Abbot's association with Croydon, and because they serve as links between the two hospitals. The statutes required these "solemn admonitions" whenever the brethren or sisters seriously misconducted themselves. "September the XVth Anno Dm̄i 1607. Robert Mason & Nicholas ffield had one & the first Admonicōn for quarrelling and fighting etc wch admonicōn was given them openly in the Chappell, in the presence of the brothers and sisters accordinge to the Statutes.

By me, Samuell ffynche, Governor, in the presence of Robt. Davies Scholemr."

" Aprill XXVth day Anno Dm̄i 1608.

Jane Meed Wydoe had one & firste Admonicōn for slaundering the foundation and state of this Hospitall. Vizt. That there are some in the house that did lyve better before they came into it etc, Openly given to her in the Chappell in the presence of the Brethren & Sisters according to the Statute.

By me Samuell ffynche, Governor.
Robt. Davies Scholemr."

" The XXVIth day of December, 1608.

Richard Hughes had one & the first Admonicōn according to the Statutes for his lewde & raylinge speaches both againste the Governors & all the whole bodie & members of the Hospitall.

Samuell ffynche Vicar.
Edwd. Burton Warden, Rob. Davies Schmr."

This is the second and last signature which Alfred Jones gives of our old friend Edward Burton.

1610. " Nycholas ffield had the seconde Admonicōn accordinge to the Statute for sowing of discorde by contentious words about the choice of the Warden to whom he himself voluntarilie gave his consenting Voice; also for slaundering governours & giving raylinge & lewde Words against others in the house. W^th the forfeite of a monthes payment . . . . given the XVth day of ffebruarij.

By Samuell ffynche Governor.

Rob. Davies.

The Warden's X marke."

Edward Burton had now died, and Robert Jenkins signs everything by his mark till he is succeeded by Jasper Yardley in 1621, except that in the last three years the schoolmaster signs for him without his mark, as if his hand or his sight had failed him. He makes his mark once more, however, in record of Yardley's election. During his 11 years of wardenship he gave " one large joyned table and a frame to the common hall " (still there), and at his death in 1626, after being a brother for 22 years, he gave £20 to the hospital.

We find an adumbration of these admonitions in the following translation from the Injunctions at St. John's Hospital, Nottingham :—

" They shall meet at least once in each week in the chapter, and excesses shall be there regularly proclaimed and corrected by the warden or master ; and the chapter shall be held without talking or noise, and those who have trangressed shall humbly and obediently undergo canonical discipline." (Clay's *Mediæval Hosp.*, p. 137.)

Samuel Fynche played so important a part in the early history of the hospital that he deserves some lines to himself. He was collated Vicar of Croydon by Archbishop Grindal on May 26th, 1581, on death of Richard Fynche. How old he was at that time we do not know, but there is collateral evidence that he was then quite a young man. Whitgift made him life-governor of his hospital, and fixed by his will (more correctly in his ordinances) a stipend for him of £6 13s. 4d., to be paid to none other acting in that capacity after his, Fynche's, death. The accounts and other entries in the ledger book are all in Fynche's beautiful and characteristic hand-writing—"court script," as Alfred Jones (incorrectly) calls it—from the beginning till July 30th, 1616. The last place where his name occurs in his own hand is of that date, at the top of a page, where we see the usual "Samuell ffynche Governour." Immediately below this comes an entry recording the expulsion of Robert Davies, Schoolmaster, and Nicholas Field, the brother whom we have already seen twice "solemnly admonished." This is undated, but in a distinctly different hand. The third from the top is in a hand different from either, and is as follows :— "Samuell Finch vicar of the parish of Croydon and overseer of this hospital deceased the 12th of September 1616." Note a capital F used to spell, not Fynche but Finch, and the term "overseer," never employed by Fynche. If we now examine the Parish Register, which begins in 1538 and has been transcribed by Mr. W. Bruce Bannerman, F.S.A., we find all the entries in the same hand from 1581, when Fynche was collated, till *and including* July 28th, 1616. The

present writer has transcribed these last several
writings as follows :—

[In margin]   " Juely
   1616   John More & Suzan Chiswicke ware
               maried the xxijth Day.
   1616   Juely
               John Batte fil. Stephani Batte was
               christened the *xxviijth Day*. (Last
               of Fynche's entries).
   1616   Juely
               Wyllm Vennar was buried the xxijth
               Day."

Immediately beneath, in a totally different hand,
as in each later case, comes the entry : " Marye Brinne
was buried the 24th daye." Three more entries follow,
then in *September* are two entries, next two words
blotted out, and below with Oct : in margin—" Samuell
Finch vicar of Croydon was buried Isth daye."

A little earlier, it was usual to bury within two days
of death, but here is an interval of 18 days, following
September 12th, when, as we have seen, he died, yet
we shall see that a whole month elapsed in the case of
Archbishop Abbot.

All this seems perfectly simple, but there intervenes
what might be mistaken as the story of another Samuel
Fynche, which appears to complicate the matter and
which, not surprisingly, puzzled Alfred Jones much.
Fynche married a girl of *fourteen* and had several
children by her, during the seven years of her married
life. On January 31st, 1582, he registered the christen-
ing of a son named Samuell, and Ducarel, in his list of

vicars of Croydon, gives these : " Samuel Fynch at the presentation of the King, by lapse, 28th February, 1603. Henry Rigge, M.A., collated by Archbishop Abbot, 20th September, 1616." Here is a complication of statements to unravel ! Who is the supposed Samuell Fynche II. ? Our authentic Samuell has, so far, a clear history. He marries early in life, has a little Samuell within a year, acts to all appearances as vicar and governor of the hospital for 35 years, and dies when at least 56 years of age.

Through the kindness, however, of Rev. Claude Jenkins, Librarian of Lambeth Palace, the mystery is practically solved. This gentleman has supplied the present writer with data from the archiepiscopal register as follows : 1. Samuel Fynche was made rector of Mongeham parva in Kent on May 27th, 1597. 2. He resigned on Jan: 27th, 1603. 3. Samuel Fynche was presented by the King to Croydon on Feb: 28th, as already stated.

As Mr. Jenkins points out, Fynche's holding both livings, unless he had a dispensation, would *de jure* create a technical vacancy at Croydon from 1597 to 1603. But we must bear in mind that Whitgift's great influence with Elizabeth might well have allowed the irregularity to be " winked at." On the accession of James I., however, this could not continue, so Fynche, presumably, resigned his rectory at Mongeham parva and was formally collated (as if *de novo*) on presentation of the King, the Archbishop being barred from acting, by statute, through lapse of time. All the while that Fynche was holding Mongeham parva and before, he was serving Whitgift at his hospital without remuneration, and he did not begin to draw his pension, as he calls it, till the Archbishop's death in February, 1603–4. This was probably the reason of Whitgift's acquiescing in the above irregularity.[1] There was, therefore, no Samuel Fynche II., in spite of the record displayed in the parish church.

A Visitation Feast.—It is interesting and amusing to note what one of the visitations cost in the way of refreshments.

For 4 chickens—2s. 0d.

  ,, 5 joints of meat—
vijs. 2d.

  ,, bread—xijd.

  ,, 2 couple of rabbits—
2s.

  ,, vinegar—2d.

  ,, spice—2d.

  ,, ginger—5d.

For oatmeal—jd.

  ,, a kilderkin of beer—
5s.

  ,, 2 quarts of sack—20d.

  ,, 2lb. of butter—xjd.

  ,, horse meat—2s.

We see no mention of vegetables. The total came to £1 3s. 7d., a much costlier repast than those provided once a year for the 30 or more brethren and sisters after 1619, when William Barlow, "sometime Bishop of Rochester," provided 13s. 4d. "for ever" for a commemoration dinner, in trust of the Fishmongers' Company. The date of this visitation was 1616, when, as a result of three adjournments, Robert Davies, schoolmaster, and Nycholas Field, brother, who, as we have seen, had already received two admonitions, were expelled. The writer has not discovered the cause of the schoolmaster's expulsion.

[1] See p. 118, as to old style dates.

A Joiner's Account.—" Payd unto Thomas Langridge the joyner the 30 of Januarye 1640 ffor setting
upp 34 yerds of Waynskott in the Chappell iijs vjd the
yerd, the guift of Mr Yardly somtyme warden of this
hospitall. ffive Pounds nineteen shillings whereof he
acknowledgeth the receite thereof as his hand hereunder showeth—V$^{l.}$ xixs more for iij dayes worke 4s. 6d.
& for 100 & 20 foote of bord to ffinish under the seates
wch cost xiiijs ijd, all is—xviijs viijd & for bread &
beare at the ffinishing of this worke—xvjd
pd for glewe for this worke and nailes wch was forgotten at the tyme wch is due unto me—xiiijd."
The total comes to £7 os. 2d.

Immediately beneath is the following—" Pd for the
makinge of the porch over the Chappell dore & the
workmanshipe & culleringe the dore & postes xxvjs."
This makes a grand total of £8 6s. 2d., and a balance
of £1 13s. 10d. out of Master Yardley's bequest of £10,
to be divided amongst the brethren and sisters. As the
artificer was illiterate, he made his mark, against
which " Thomas Langridge his marke " is written by
another's hand. This porch to the chapel appears to
have been now made for the first time.

Bede Gowns.—No mention is made in Whitgift's
statutes of costume, though the inmates had to attend
the parish church marching " orderlye by two and two
together " on Sundays, festivals, etc. It appears, however, that £30 was spent every two years on gowns, and,
as we saw in the footnote (p. 113), Edward Aylworth
gave 26 gowns. From a letter transcribed in the ledger
book dated October 29th, 1681, and addressed, not to
the warden but to John Cæsar the defaulting school-

master, we gather that the wearing of gowns at church had been neglected during the Commonwealth and that the inmates were not to "presume" to appear there save in the habit of the hospital.

Inventory of 1634.—"In the Treasury, two stronge chestes, a table, a courte Cubbard, a chaire, a joynte stool, in one of the chestes all the Evidences & leases of lands, in the other a broade bowle of silver and gilt [Dean Neville's], a greate standinge Cuppe of wodd tipt with sylver [Parker's], a little silver cuppe for wine [since gone], a mazer tipt with silver and gilt, the seale of Hospitall."

"In the audience chamber, A faire drawinge table [*i.e.*, with leaf which could be drawn out], 18 joyned stools, the portrait of the Founder," &c.

Of the nineteen "joyned stools" mentioned in the hospital, but one remains. (See Figs. 20, 21 and 22.)

There is no later Inventory, but an earlier one is dated 1601, and therein the mazer "tipt with silver," which is that shown in Fig. 24, is mentioned, although not appearing in the list of benefactions, as of Mr. Boulton's gift. It would likely weary the general reader were we to quote these inventories at any length, and we need only note a few more points. Whitgift's Hospital was abundantly supplied from the first with ordinary domestic stuff, much of which, as we have seen, was given by friends, pewter holding a considerable proportion and weighing nearly two stone. Of these things a few pewter "chargers" and delf-ware dishes still remain. A few more articles of finer quality, such as cushions, coverlets, glass-ware, &c., are mentioned, and most of them (not the fabrics) were kept in the Treasury, only to be brought out, apparently, on state occasions. Another " courte cubbard " besides that in the Treasury is mentioned, and is now in the warden's sitting room.

Whitgift's Arms.—The Whitgift family not being territorial, John, on his elevation to the bishopric of Worcester, had a grant of arms. This matter is fully discussed by C. S. Percival in the *Surrey Archæological Collections*, Vol. II. In accordance with invariable rule handed down from ancient times, the archbishop of Canterbury's personal arms are impaled with those of the See. That is to say, in the dexter half (opposite the right of the warrior as he bore his shield in front of him) there is displayed, on a *blue* ground, the Archiepiscopal Pallium or emblem of the actual vestment given by the Pope, in pre-Reformation days. This is represented as *silver* edged and fringed with *gold* and charged (bearing upon it) four small *black* crosses tapered at the lower end. Behind, and nearly hidden by the pallium, is a *gold* bishop's staff " ensigned " with a cross of the same. Whitgift's first grant of arms was described as, on a *gold* (or) ground, a *blue* flowered (flory) cross charged with *four* bezants. The bezant in British heraldry is an ancient charge representing the Byzantine gold coins with which it is supposed the higher soldiers in the holy wars were paid, and is, therefore, always blazoned *or*. There were various modifications in Whitgift's personal arms as time went on, but they were always on the sinister side of his shield. The final form, and alone seen in his hospital, was *Silver*, a cross flory *sable*, with *five* bezants *or*. These have been spoken of as representing the five stigmata of Christ and so they may have been considered by Whitgift in his later years. He was also granted a crest —a ducal coronet with a lion's paw proceeding from it and holding a green laurel wreath—but there is no evidence of his ever having used it, although it is painted, probably at a later date, upon one of his portraits in Lambeth Palace, as will presently be seen.

In one of the windows of the hall, as we have seen, there is a crown in amber glass, which might be taken carelessly for a ducal coronet but is not, the representation being the same as that on Queen Elizabeth's head in the picture at the Houses of Parliament. It is remarkable that on a scroll beneath this crown is the motto—" vincit qui patitur," nowhere else seen in the hospital, but recognised as Whitgift's and placed beneath his arms with the *four* bezants in Sir George Paule's Life of the archbishop. Mottoes are not the exclusive property of the users, and this particular motto appears attached to the arms of the Chester family in West Surrey and to several others. It has been said that it " reads both ways," but how this can be is not obvious, unless we say, with some truth, that while he conquers who endures or suffers, he who conquers suffers. (" Some victories are worse than defeats.") We know that Edward Aylworth, Whitgift's friend, paid for the original glass in the hall, and it is likely that both wished to perpetuate the memory of Whitgift's indebtedness to Elizabeth by associating his motto with her personal crown.

The archiepiscopal mitre is seen on the hospital buildings and on documents of the Whitgift Foundation with a ducal coronet, but A. C. Fox Davies, in his *Art of Heraldry*, 1904, says that the mitres of archbishops and bishops are properly the same, except that of the Bishop of Durham, who alone is entitled to surround his with a ducal coronet in virtue of the ancient palatine rights of his see.

Portraits of Whitgift.—In Croydon Public Library there are a number of prints and photographs, collected by the late Rev. H. J. Clayton, representing authentic portraits of Whitgift in various places and at different ages. Twelve of these may be selected as illustrating the aspects of the man in successive periods of his life arranged, so far as can be ascertained, according to age.

1. In Peterhouse College, Cambridge, dated 1560, when he had been a fellow five years and was then 30. He received his first preferment in that year, on taking orders, but is represented merely in academic dress.

2. A full-length portrait in University College, Durham. No date or age are shown, but, as he appears in episcopal garb with full black beard without any trace of grey hairs, it is safe to assume that he was then Bishop of Worcester and at least 47 years of age.

3. A photograph of a picture in Lambeth Palace without date or age, but with Whitgift's personal arms showing *five bezants* surmounted by helmet mantling and the crest described on p. 131. The left-hand fingers are inserted into a book, and the beard is as black as in the Durham portrait. The first grant of a crest was in 1588, and that of the fifth bezant in 1598. The portrait hardly represents a man of 58, as Whitgift would have been in 1588, and certainly not 68, when he was presumably entitled to five bezants. It seems,

PLATE XIV.

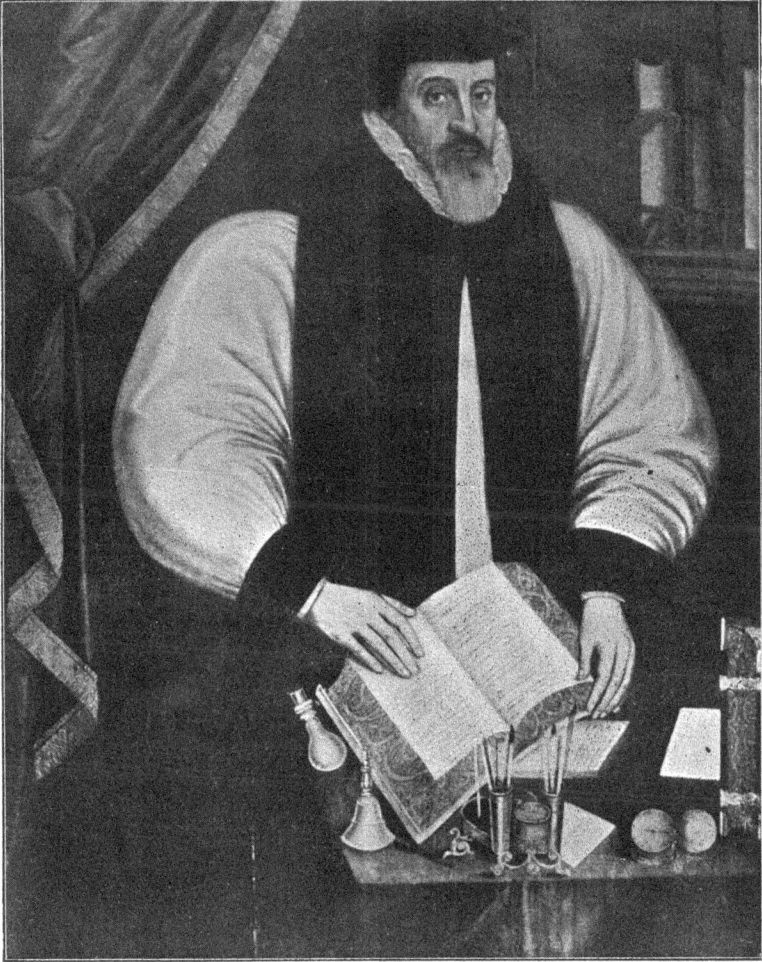

Fig. 25.—PORTRAIT OF WHITGIFT IN CHAPEL
By permission of Mrs Streatfield

[*Face p. 132*

therefore, a fair inference that this heraldic device was painted in at some later date, and that the picture was made when the original was considerably younger, possibly while still Bishop of Worcester.

4. In Trinity College, Cambridge : no date or age, but the beard streaked with grey.

5. A coloured lithograph with Whitgift's full arms showing five bezants, his motto *Vincit qui patitur*, without crest, above 1602 and below AET 68.   Close under the print appears " printed in Holland," while the legend reads " By permission of his Grace the Archbishop of Canterbury, from the original picture in Lambeth Palace."   The date and age given are incompatible with each other, for in 1602 Whitgift was 72. He is curiously represented here with a *golden* beard and hazel eyes—never his colouring—and the general appearance is that of a man scarcely more than 60.

6. A portrait in the University Library at Cambridge. AET 68 is in one corner, there are abundant grey hairs, and the picture might well represent a man of that age.

7. Save for minor details, the undated portrait in the chapel at Croydon might be a copy of 6, yet the face is not quite so severe or aggressive.   See Fig. 25.

8. A painting in the National Portrait Gallery without date or age.   It looks more artistic than Nos. 6 and 7, but seems of about the same age.

9. A painting which appears much obscured, but might be a copy of that in Cambridge Library, in Archdeacon Plume's Library at Malden.

10. Portrait at Lambeth Palace, undated, with full white beard, but lacking the individuality of all the other authentic portraits.

K

11. A very quaint series of engravings quite unlike the preceding, from a portrait formerly at Lambeth but since missing. One of these was used as a frontispiece to Sir George Paule's *Life of Whitgift*, shows *five* bezants, and his age 73 at death, as if it were the final portrait.

12. A picture at Knole in Kent. This, though by an unknown painter, is the most artistic of the series. Here we see an old man in whose face the seriousness remains, but the austerity has disappeared, who in his serenity can contemplate the joy of providing that, for a few poor people at least, " at evening time it shall be light."

End of Corporate Life.—Alfred Jones writes :— " From first to last the Corporation of the Hospital was seldom free from a suit at law, generally at a disadvantage, and especially during the first twenty years of the nineteenth century." In 1820 we read of Mr. Drummond, of Croydon, being appointed solicitor by the corporation of the hospital in place of Mr. Edwards, whose charges were excessive. But the brethren found their last case worse than their first, for Mr. Drummond's regulating ended in loss of their status as a corporation of freeholders. Placed by the Charity Commission under a board of Governors, a long system of curtailments ensued whereby all their back land was lost to them, a limited portion of the vast revenues of the " Whitgift Foundation " ear-marked for the Hospital. The rest goes to the Schools (no longer Whitgift's Free School) to which they, their founder's " brothers and sisters," but now the Charity Commission's " alms people," are themselves an annex.

There is much in this charming old building that appeals to the antiquarian, to the person of taste, and to the artistic draughtsman and photographer, but the writer's advice to his readers would be—" Go and see for yourselves," as indeed many do from all quarters of the world, including even some of the townspeople of **Croydon.**

CHAPTER XIII

TRINITY HOSPITAL AT GUILDFORD

GUILDFORD and Croydon have some resemblances, but many and more marked differences. Both were Anglo-Saxon settlements at the northern foot of the chalk uplands of Surrey, through which, of old time, the Wey and the Wandle, each arising where is now the Weald, had each cut its channel. Yet these two towns have had very distinctive histories and developments.

Guildford,[1] by the ford of its river, grew to be an important market-town, and the official capital of the county. It belonged to Alfred the Great, and was a royal borough and a stronghold from early times. The castle keep is Norman, the church of St. Mary retains pre-Conquest portions in its fabric, and there are some quaint old streets and many old houses.

Croydon, the Anglo-Saxon *Crogden* or the place in the *crooked valley*, chosen by our forefathers for the abundance of its springs, remained for many centuries a village, unimportant save for the country residence of the archbishops of Canterbury, and for charcoal-burning at the edge of the great North Wood. Yet it has grown, especially during the past forty years, into

---

[1] The *ford* in Gyldeford or Geldeford, as in Shalford, a little higher up stream, is beyond question, but the qualifying prefix is of doubtful origin. Three solutions have been offered. 1. *geld*, a toll. The junction of several trade-routes would make the place important, perhaps from pre-historic days. 2. *geleht*, wet—the liability to flooding about here would often render the approaches to the ford marshy. 3. Patronymic.

a vast modern town of thronged streets and of residences joining it to London, for which, in fact, it serves largely as a dormitory.   Still, both places have this in common, that each had its pre-Reformation hospital, for in Croydon Ely Davy, whose memorial brass is in the parish church, built a small almshouse in the time of Henry VI., succeeded by a modern edifice serving the same purpose, while Guildford has but the memory of the thirteenth-century hospital of St. Thomas, retained in comparatively recent times by the name " Spital Street " till it was replaced by another deemed more euphonious.

As there are likenesses and differences between Croydon and Guildford, so were there between John Whitgift and his successor (after the brief primacy of Bancroft), George Abbot.   The fathers of both were men of mercantile engagements, both were Protestants of Geneva type, both became ecclesiastics in early life, and each *founded an important hospital during his lifetime*.   But here the resemblance ends.   Whitgift, throughout his episcopacy, was strenuously occupied with setting on a firm basis the Anglican Church in accordance with the political views of Queen Elizabeth. Abbot came into his high office in the reign of James I., when that organisation was more firmly established. He did, indeed, accomplish a measure of approximation between Scottish Presbyterianism and English Prelacy, but such controversies as engaged him were rather with Roman Catholics than with the Brownists or Separatists of Whitgift's days.   Indeed, though Abbot had not the strong leanings towards Puritanism which led to the suspension of Grindal by Elizabeth, he was accused by his enemies of being too lenient with Protestant dissenters, while Whitgift was charged by the Separatists with being more tolerant of Papists than of them.

In personal character, there was considerable dissimilarity between these two men. Whitgift, while he magnified his office, moving from place to place with a large retinue, and requiring service on bended knee, seems to have deemed this due to " John of Canterbury." As " John Whitgift " he thought himself of little consequence ; he would not take office, though Elizabeth wished it, while Edmund Grindal lived, and it is said of him that on occasions when the Queen honoured him with her presence he would go to Croydon and dwell among his poor at his hospital. In that place there is scarce visible a trace of John Whitgift's personality ; no attempts at grandeur and but little ornament. All expenditure was directed to the greatest happiness of the greatest possible number. Whitgift was, as has been said, no man of affairs, showed an almost child-like trust in the good faith of his own " cloth," and and appears to have believed in a degree of democracy, with disastrous results.

Abbot was the better scholar, and was one of the translators of the New Testament in the authorised version. His character seems to have been " more of a piece " than Whitgift's, for while he does not appear set on " magnifying his office " there is no more evidence than in Whitgift of desire for personal exaltation. The style of his hospital, less " fitting " than that of Whitgift, and the frequent repetition therein of the words— *Clamamus Abba Pater*," We cry ' our Father '," which looks like a play on his own name, might seem opposed to the idea of self-effacement. Yet it must be borne in mind that while Whitgift provided in the town of his adoption, not of his birth, like Great Grimsby, for a large district, Abbot erected a hospital in the place where he had been born, where he went to school, where his parents had lived before him, and where there was then no House of Pity. To build one worthy of Guildford must be taken as a praiseworthy ambition. Of this he himself laid the foundation-stone on April 6th, 1619. As to the words quoted, the so-called *pun* on his own name may have been quite unconscious. They certainly express Abbot's consistent belief in the doctrine of Election, and were meant as a reminder to the inmates and to typify to them the teaching, for they came not there by right of their own but by the considered choice of their governors.

Abbot, though, like Whitgift, he enjoyed the friendship of his sovereign, James I., throughout his primacy, showed his independence by more than once opposing the wishes of the Court. This brought upon him the dislike of no less powerful personages than Charles, Laud, and the Duke of Buckingham. This and his grief at accidentally killing a keeper while out hunting, at the age of sixty, led to his retirement to Guildford and Croydon, at which latter place he died on August 4th, 1633, when aged seventy-one.

The Burial Certificate of Archbishop Abbot is transcribed in Vol. III. of the *Surrey Archæological Collections*. His " Funeralls " were " most honourably solemnised " at Croydon on September 3rd—one month, be it noted, after his death. Amongst the notabilities who attended was Abbot's quondam antagonist, not to say enemy, Laud, now Archbishop designate, and Sir Charles Cæsar, Master of the Rolls. The procession then passed on its way to Guildford, where it was met by the Mayor and Corporation, while the obsequies were ordered and attended by Sir Wm. Segar, Garter or Principal King of Arms (he who in 1599 subscribed Whitgift's Charter of Incorporation as " Norroy King of Armes "), Sir Richard St. George, Clarencieux King of Arms, Sir John Borough, Norroy King of Arms, and Richmond and Lancaster Heralds. The document is subscribed as correct by Maurice (or Morris) Abbot, his brother, and George Abbot, his nephew.

Abbot's residence in Croydon a little earlier than the hunting catastrophe is attested by the following entries in the Ledger-books extracted by Alfred Jones. Under " Solemn Admonitions," according to Whitgift's statutes are these :—

"March 3 1617. The above named Maurice Powell was convented before my Lord's Grace of Canterbury, [Abbot], in the greate Chamber at the place [Palace] of Croydon, Sir Robert Hatton, Steward, Mr. Scott, Treasurer and divers others of his Grace's gentlemen then present, for like disorder, viz. : gaming, drinking and rayling, and was then lessoned, persuaded and threatened, to amend his disordered life. It was, therefore, by his Grace there enacted that when any of the like disorders should be againe proved against the above mentioned Maurice Powell, he should then Ipso facto be displaced and removed the Hospitall."

" Nov. 3 1619. Roger Pinson had a solemn 2nd admonition given him by my Lord's Grace of Canter-burye in his greate chamber at the place of Croydon for denying my Lord's Grace his Authoritye in the Hospitall. Sr. Robert Hatton, Mr. Scott &c being present. It was then also enacted that upon the next disorder he shall be displaced & removed from the Hospitall." Corbet Anderson, in his *Chronicle of Croydon*, says Abbot resided much at Croydon and quotes the Harleian MSS. on the point.

The Master, not styled " Warden," at Guildford, was to be chosen as a *man of business capacity*, especially as regarded landed property, by five electors, namely, the Mayor of Guildford, the Parson of Holy Trinity Church, the Vice-master and the two eldest Brethren, and he was not necessarily a poor brother. There was no chaplain, the master himself conducting the daily services in the chapel. In fact, the influence of the minor clergy was not great at Guildford Hospital. This clearly shows Abbot's better business capacity and knowledge of men. On the other hand, while Samuel Fynche acted as governor at Croydon, so long as he was vicar, and Whitgift begged his successors in general terms to have supervision, Abbot placed this more directly in the hands of the Archbishops. There was no need for him to make provision for free education at Guildford, because the free Grammar-school had long previously existed in that town. His business sympathies are also shown by his devoting part of his endowments to encouraging manufacture in Guildford.

Abbot's Statutes are dated 1629, ten years after his hospital was founded, and signed : *G. Cant* in presence of Sir Morris (or Maurice) Abbot, his younger brother; Maurice Abbot, his nephew; Ric : Brigham, his controller ; and Walter

Dobson, his receiver. **George Abbot died** as we have seen, at
Croydon in 1633 and was buried in Holy Trinity Church
at Guildford, where his tomb remains as erected by
Sir Maurice. Over a recumbent effigy in white marble,
a canopy is reared supported by four pillars of black
and two of mottled marble, while two more are seen at
the back. Several emblematic figures represent the
conceptions of Edmund Spenser, whose Canto X.,
quoted as our opening lines, evidently inspired the
designer.

George Abbot's Arms.—Unlike John Whitgift, George
Abbot was descended from a territorial family, and, as
a younger son, was entitled to a coat of arms with a
difference, namely, *Gules*, a Chevron between three
pears, *Or*, with a Mullet (representing the rowel of a
spur) of the first for difference. Maurice, the son next
to George, had a martlet for difference.

Inspection of the Hospital.—We may now explore
the famous Hospital of the Blessed Trinity, which stands
imposingly on the north side of the High Street of
Guildford, its great outer gate-house with four angle-
turrets forming a conspicuous landmark from a distance.
Here is a Jacobean not an Elizabethan edifice, the Tudor
quality not being in evidence, save for the fireplaces and
some doorways and doors. We miss the rustic touch
and relative spaciousness prevailing in Croydon, but
the rear grounds, filched away from Whitgift's Hospital,
are represented at Guildford by a large garden on the
north side, from which, indeed, the best idea of the
extension of the buildings can be obtained. The
Master's quarters, entered from a porch in the south-

Plate XV.

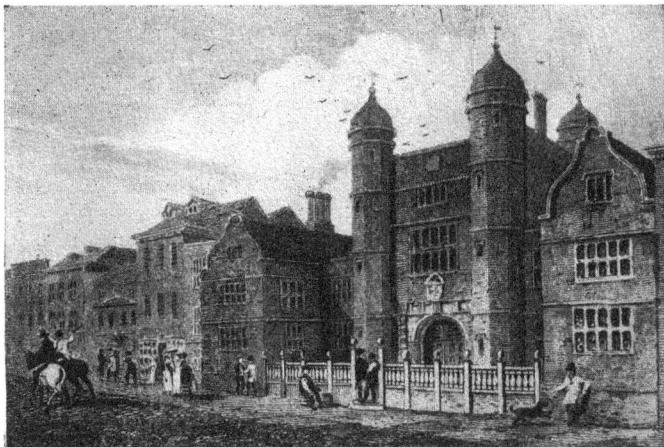

Fig. 26.—TRINITY HOSPITAL, GUILDFORD,
IN 19th CENTURY

By permission of the Master

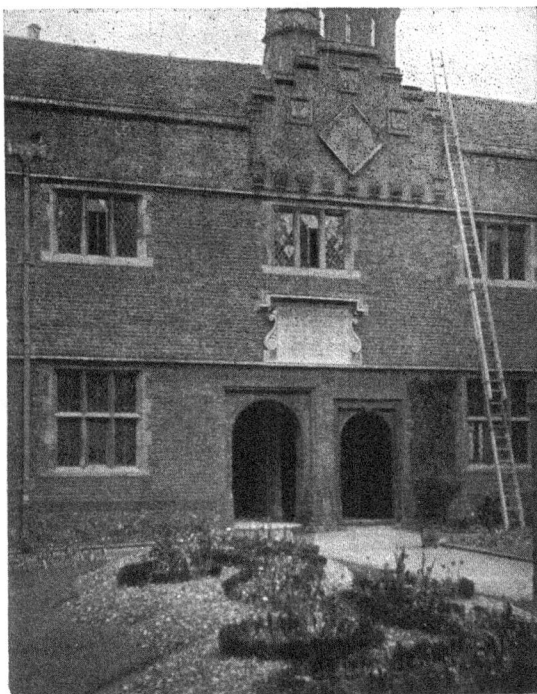

Fig. 27.—NORTH SIDE OF QUADRANGLE

[Face p. 142

east of the quadrangle, are contiguous with and originally included the Presence Chamber, now the Board-
room, in the Gate-house, with the muniment-room above
and contain a beautiful carved staircase, very unlike
the narrow flight of steps to the Warden's rooms at
Croydon. The chimney-stacks of varied form, with
their distinct flues, are particularly fine examples of
brick-work. In the north-east of the quadrangle is
the entrance to the Chapel, where are two great windows
in the east and north respectively filled with original
stained-glass portraying the story of Jacob with Latin
commentaries beneath. The brethren on the west and
the sisters on the east have each a single room ; there
are no married couples, but there are quarters, absent
at Croydon, for a nurse. The outstanding feature of an
inner gate-house is not at once noticed as at Croydon, but
a central archway leading to the garden marks a correspondence. High in this face are displayed the arms of
the See of Canterbury, the initials G.A., and Abbot's
personal arms, in this case showing the mullet difference.
We may observe here, too, some chevron ornament in
brick—a curious incongruity one would think, amidst
Renaissance work. On the right of the archway we see
the door and casements of the Common Hall, and above
is the old Guest-room or " Greate Chamber." This is
reached by a wide staircase ascending in two flights
from a carved wooden arch within the building.

To the student of English life in this period of
transition from the Mediæval to the Modern, these
likenesses and unlikenesses between Whitgift's Hospital
and her slightly younger sister at Guildford are very
interesting. Both are dedicated to the Trinity, Abbot

substituting " Blessed " for " Holy." In fact, long before, in his commentaries on the Prophet Jonah, Abbot was very emphatic in condemning what he called invocations of saints, saying if one dedicates a place it should be to God alone. Yet, whether Whitgift and he knew it or no, several very ancient hospitals were dedicated to the Saviour or to the Trinity, as a review will show us.

Amongst other links between the two hospitals we may note this. Edward Aylworth, the friend of Whitgift, who gave those " xxvj rugg gownes " to Croydon at his death, left by his will " twentie black rugg Gownes " to the smaller community at Guildford. These were received on December 7th, 1626, and, as the complement of brothers and sisters was made up in that year, these must have been their first uniforms, though later and ever since they have been of a dark blue. Uniforms have long been extinct at Croydon, but not so at Guildford, where they are worn both by brothers and sisters at daily prayers in chapel, on going in procession to church over the way, by the brother who takes his turn as porter, and by the Master when he attends Board-meetings, &c. There are silver badges attached, bearing the insignia of the founder and handed down by each to his successor. We shall presently notice these again.

James I.'s letters patent, or Charter, are kept framed in the Presence Chamber, not stored away in a strong-room as at Croydon, and have somewhat lost the colour of the illuminations. It is so like Elizabeth's to Croydon that, *mutatis mutandis*, it might be taken for a copy. King James's bust appears within his initial J,

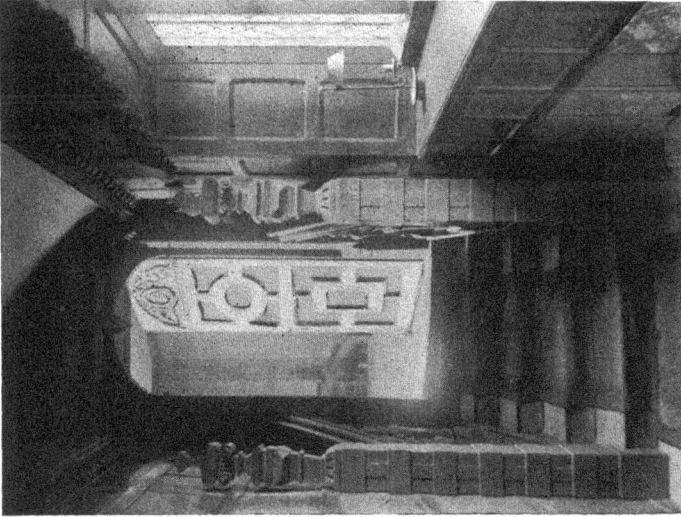

Fig. 28.—ENTRANCE TO PRESENCE CHAMBER

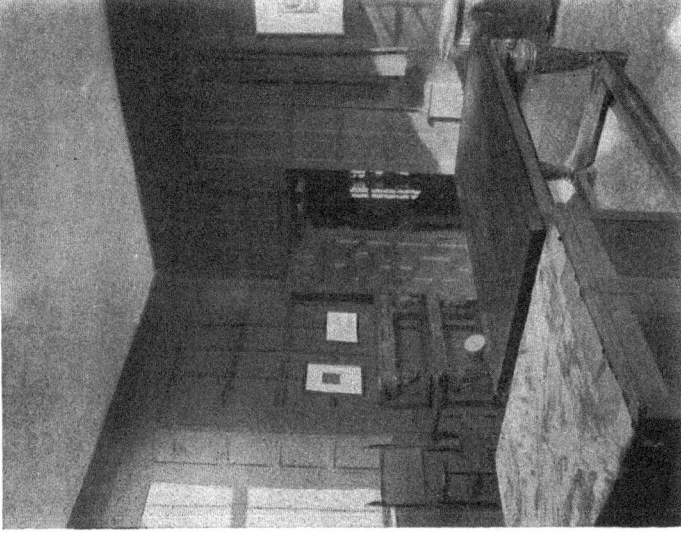

Fig. 29.—PRESENCE CHAMBER

[*Face p. 144*

crowned on the top of his hat ! He claims kingship of Scotland (to which Elizabeth did not in her charter lay any claim), of France, and of *unimportant* Ireland, besides, of course, England. There are some slight differences in the upper border; the crowned and bearded lion (or is it a leopard ?) still supports the flag with the red cross of St. George, but the Queen's dragon is evidently being " evolved " into a unicorn, and is holding the St. Andrew's saltire cross of Scotland.

The round seal of Guildford is wholly different from that of Croydon. In heraldic fashion, Archbishop Abbot's arms are displayed, surmounted by an epis-copal mitre, and supported by a man and a woman in dresses too sumptuous for the " rugg gownes " of the beneficiaries, between whose heads is a scroll bearing Abbot's favourite " motto," *Clamamus Abba Pater.*

For the sake of comparison with Whitgift's Hospital, and to throw additional " side-lights " on contemporary life in the seventeenth century, a few extracts are given from an article by Mr. Philip G. Palmer, Master, on *Inventories of 1633 and Later.*[1] The article is based on the entries of Jasper Yardley, second Master, during nine years, who, as we have seen, left Whitgift's to take up the mastership at Guildford, and this inventory is a year earlier than the second one at the elder hospital.

" Imprimis in the Chappell.

A greate Bible bossed, a Service booke, Six Saulters & our ffounders Armes fairely done & hanged up ther, a long brush." The Bible, etc. have, Mr. Palmer tells us, long since disappeared unrecorded. The

[1] *Surrey Arch. Coll.,* Vol. XXX.

arms constituted the hatchment brought thither after the archbishop's funeral, which has remained there ever since ; the mullet difference is duly displayed ; Sir Maurice Abbot was at the cost of making, but the hospital paid 1s. porterage.

" Item in the greate Chamber.

A picture of my Lord our ffounder. A large drawing Table, a Court cupbord & one Dozen of Joynt Stooles. Sir Nicholas Kempes Picture." Sir Nicholas was a notable benefactor ; Abbot's portraits will receive attention later. The joint or joined stools were more solidly built than those at Croydon and consequently more have survived, but the guilloche ornament on the one forlorn representative there and on the overmantel is entirely absent at Guildford. The " court cupbord " has disappeared, but Croydon is more fortunate in retaining one with its beautiful hinges in a corner of the Warden's room.

" Item in XX^{tie} Chambers for the brothers and sisters.

XX^{tie} halfe headed Bedsteds." Some of these were afterwards lent to the " lower hospital " for outside sick folk. This replaced the " Manufacture " established by Abbot and was itself superseded by Archbishop Abbot's School, founded with his funds upon the remnants of Baker's Elizabethan Bluecoat School in 1860. Mr. Palmer says *fortunately* these do not seem to have been returned. Doubtless, they were wooden.

" Item in the Treasury [Muniment room].

A little Table, Two greate Chests, one for ye Hospitall, the other for the Manufacture, a Cabinet

with boxes in w^chˡ are the wriytings, The Charter of
the house, the booke of Statutes, The Comon Seale of
brasse, Two silver Boles, a greate and a lesse, Two
silver Saultes a greate & a lesse, & two dozen of silver
Spoones, one lesse, the other greater." The common
seal is already described. The plate is further
alluded to in the inventories of 1709 and 1749. The
" boles " were evidently mazers, and we learn that
the larger held about 2 quarts, the smaller about one
quart—doubtless for the ladies. We may be sure
that the fine things here enumerated were kept for
" Gaudy Days," such as the four annual feasts, to wit,
Christmas, Easter, Whitsuntide and the Founder's
Birthday—October 29th, old style. In 1764 all this
plate, except four silver spoons, was sold, being so
much dead stock, " with the Consente and approba-
tion of all the rest of the Brethren " (that of the sisters
was not required, not being of the corporation) and
£36 11s. 1d. realised. Unfortunately we know
nothing of the hall-marks on the mazers, and therefore cannot tell their dates. The four unsold spoons
are kept in the Presence Chamber, and bear hall-
marks variously of 1608–9, 1624–5 and 1669–70. The
little table, the two chests, the book of Statutes,
the cabinet, the containing boxes are all in the
hospital.

Says Mr. Palmer : " This [the statute book] is a hand-
some manuscript of vellum, bound in whole calf, with
brass corners and clasps, the Founder's Arms stamped
in gold upon each cover. The Statutes are signed by
the Founder." The little boxes contained the title

deeds, and were just the same as those at Croydon, even to the lining with printer's waste paper.

" A bell to ring to prayers in one turret." This was changed in 1662 for another bell weighing 15½ lbs.— an instrument very different from the little hand-bell at Whitgift's Hospital for the same purpose.

Mr. Palmer says that the Porter's Lodge mentioned in the inventory was on the west side of the garden entrance, and that the door of it was originally two-leaved horizontally. This antique arrangement may still be seen in the kitchen premises at Croydon Palace, and some old country cottages. Probably the intent was to allow of parley, without giving too easy access to strangers.

The Archbishop did not hesitate to censure his brother Richard, the first Master. Thus : " My lo^d is informed yo^u make his Hospitall a store house for Corne & is much displeased wth it, therfore yo^u must not suffer it."

Respecting badges on the gowns ; there are two entries in the ledger-book of date 1745 : " Apl. 12 Paid ffor 3 Mitter y^e Lord Bisshops Armes 01.17.10." Then later, " Paid Mr. Medden for Mending a Mittre 6$^{d.}$" Note the archaic spelling still surviving. Mitter or mittre means the badge which is a bishop's mitre. Of these silver badges, the master's is slightly larger than the rest, which are worn by the brethren and not by the sisters. Eight of the original have been preserved and there are now 14 in all. Material for the gowns cost 4s. 6d. the yard in 1630–33. The making up of these cost 1s. 6d. each in 1633 and 1638, and was a bi-yearly expense. Mr. Williamson, in his book mentioned

PLATE XVII.

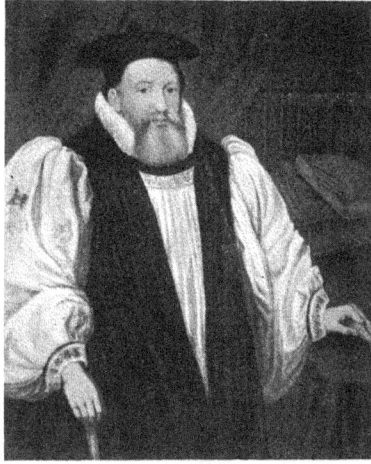

Fig. 30.—PORTRAIT OF ARCHBISHOP ABBOT

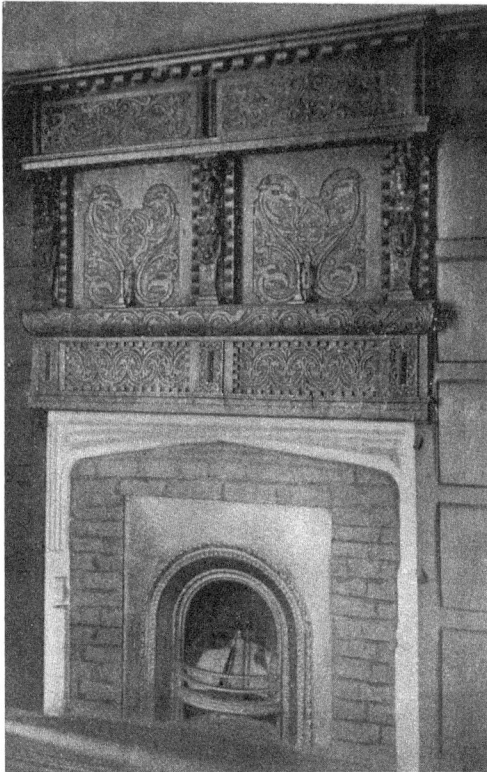

Fig. 31.—OVER-MANTEL IN MASTER'S QUARTERS

[Face p. 148

below, quotes from the ledger book—" 1632, Sept. 8th Paid to Goodman John West for IX waine loades of Charrcoles att xxj^s pr loade and wood in all 10,00,00." " Paid for a Christmas Days dinner for us all xs."

The Founder's Portrait now hangs in the Presence Chamber. It has been several times restored, and an expert considered it had somewhat suffered thereby. It bears date 1623, and is conjectured to be the work of a scholar of Paul van Somer, but there is no record from whence it came. It is copied in Speaker Onslow's *Life of Abbot.* Mr. G. C. Williamson reproduces another portrait of George Abbot in his book, *Guildford in the Olden Time,* says it was of about 1618, the work of Cornelius Janssens, and gives the history of its coming into his possession from Croydon Palace, where it had previously hung.[1]   There are also portraits in the presence chamber of Sir Nicholas Kempe, of Ald. Jackman, another benefactor, and of the reformers John Wycliff, John Foxe, John Calvin and Sebastian Menster. These seem to emphasise George Abbot's sympathies. It is very curious that the name *Abbot* induces in the minds of some visitors the vague idea of a monastic building, a conception so much the reverse of the founder's tone of thought that the present Master resents the appellation " Abbot's Hospital," and is emphatic in using the real name of the place, " The Hospital of the Blessed Trinity." It has suffered far less from restoration than the Hospital of the Holy Trinity at Croydon, and though a much finer building,

---

[1] In Croydon Public Library is a print of Archbishop Abbot, engraved by W. T. Mote, " from the original in the collection of the Rt. Hon. the Earl of Verulam." There is no date, but the portrait is a pleasing one, evidently painted when Abbot was quite an old man.   See Fig. 30.

L

a " museum of Jacobean art " one may fairly call it, yet, in the author's eyes, Whitgift's Hospital, partly perhaps from long familiarity with it, seems the more beautiful. But he would say to his readers—Go yourselves to these two sister Houses of Pity, see, learn and judge for yourselves. They stand not very far apart nor far from London.

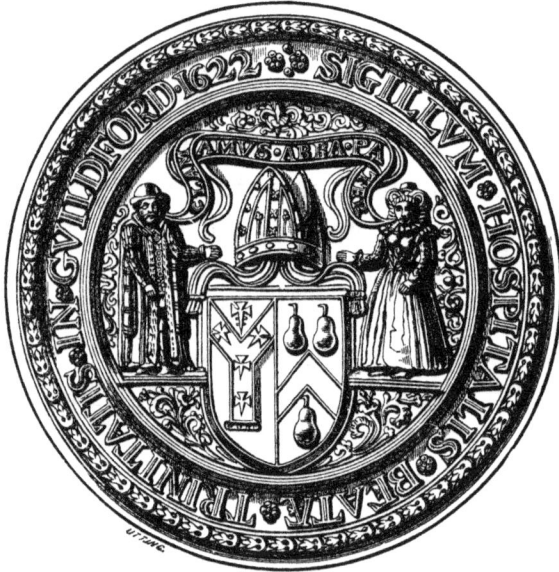

FIG. 33.—SEAL OF HOSPITAL,

By permission of Surrey Archæological Society.

PLATE XVIII.

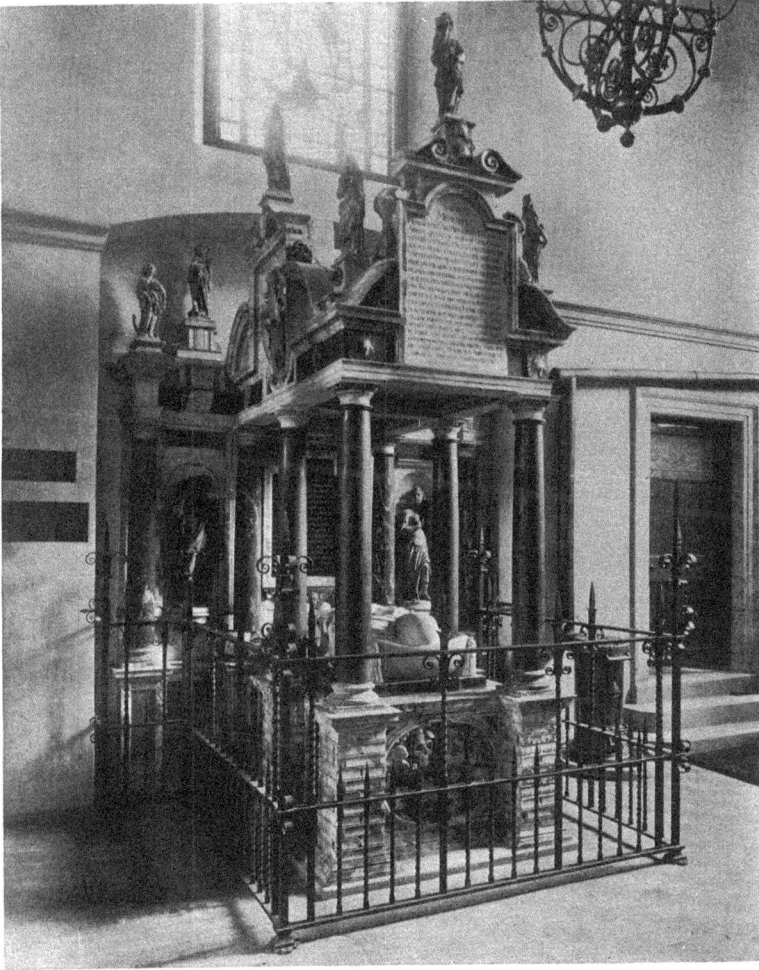

Fig. 32.—ARCHBISHOP ABBOT'S TOMB

By permission of Mr P. G. Palmer, Master

[*Face p. 150*

CHAPTER XIV

LONDON NORTH OF THE THAMES

Knights of St. John.—Nearly fifty years before the first Crusade of 1096–7, *i.e.*, in 1045, certain Benedictine monks established a hospital in Jerusalem for relief of pilgrims to the Holy Places who had been wounded, robbed, or fallen sick. Their first patron saint was John, patriarch of Alexandria, who, in the sixth century, when the Saracens first took Jerusalem, sent money and goods to the Christians in Syria. Later, the monks renounced their original saint—not an isolated instance—in favour of St. John the Baptist, who, as a wanderer, was in high esteem for a patron of pilgrim-houses, and, as we have seen abundantly, of hospitals. Soon after the first Crusade, these monks formed themselves into a military order, and were henceforth known as the Knights of St. John at Jerusalem, or the Knights Hospitallers. For several centuries these fighting monks were an extraordinary power—a kingdom within the kingdoms of Europe—but they never lost their original character of tenders of the ailing and wounded. When finally driven to Malta by the Turks, they made it their headquarters and stronghold, and were henceforth known as the Knights of Malta. Their vast hospital on that island survives to the present day, and was much used during the Great War. The writer remembers, as a child of five, seeing at Malta the stone stairs with very low rises, up which the knights were wont to ride. The Maltese cross, their badge, is a modification of the Greek cross. It has four equal limbs, expanding outwards and forked at the end. (See p. 50, Chap. VI.) The Hospitallers had their Priory at Clerkenwell, founded in 1100 by Jordan Briset, knight or baron, where they remained till suppressed at the Dissolution. The heads of the house were styled " Lord Prior," and took precedence of all lay barons in Parliament. During the Peasants' Rising, in 1381, the buildings were burned down and Lord Prior Dowcra rebuilt them, the gate-house known as Dowcra's gate and still spanning the street being the last of his work, finished in 1504. Amongst the several benefactors to the Priory, Roger de Mowbray, whose name we have met with on p. 11, as the founder of Burton Lazars, was the chief. At the Dissolution, Henry VIII. granted the site to John, Viscount Lisle, and in the third year of Edward VI. a great part of the chapel was blown up. Phillip and Mary in greater part restored the order, but it was finally suppressed by Elizabeth. So long as Henry lived, the place was kept from spoil, being used as a store for sporting and military purposes. James I. granted the south, or Dowcra's gate, to Sir Roger Wilbraham for his lifetime, and other portions came into the hands of various proprietors. Nothing remains of Dowcra's building or those of earliest date save his gate-house and the Norman crypt beneath the comparatively modern chapel, on some stones of which the present writer has seen the masons' marks.

A latter-day revival of the order is known as St. John's Ambulance Association, and has its headquarters on the site.

St. Anthony's, once on the north side of Threadneedle Street, in the City, had its origin in a Jewish Synagogue. John Stowe, who wrote as a contemporary of its last phase of decadence in 1598, has these facts to tell us of St. Anthony's. The Jews' Synagogue was built about 1231, and Henry III., upon their displacement and transfer of the place to the Fraternity of St. Anthony in France, dedicated it to the Virgin. A hospital being " since " established, was called St. Anthony's, and portions of land *subsequently* given afforded sites for a large free school and almshouses. It is evident from this that the poor had previously been received into the original hospital, and that the religious staff remained there. Henry VI. gave the master and brethren several endowments towards the maintenance of scholars who were first to be instructed in the rudiments of grammar at Eton College, of his foundation, and then to pass to the Faculty of Arts at Oxford, each receiving 10d. per week. Five years later, *viz.*, in 1447, the Pope allowed entire severance from the old parent house at Vienne, while in 1474 Edward IV. granted to the master to have priests, clerks, scholars, poor men and brethren " of the same," choristers, proctors, etc., similarly to the foreign convent—evidently a new charter. He also " annexed, united and appropriated " the foundation to the Collegiate Church of St. George at Windsor. The hospital was " in being " in 1529, for Stowe tells us that Walter Chapman gave £20 to the " bedemen," but its annexation to Windsor led to its eventual extinction. A former schoolmaster named Johnson, when he became prebend of that church (no date given), " by little and little followed the spoil of the Hospitall : first he dissolved the Quire, conveyed [away] the plate and ornaments, then the bels and lastly put out the Almsmen from their houses, appointing them portions of twelve pence the weeke to each (but now I hear of no such performed) ; their houses with other be letten out for rent, and the Church is a preaching place for the French nation." The once famous school had come to nothing in Stowe's time.

He tells us of disputes leading to fights in the streets between the boys of St. Paul's and St. Anthony's, the first being dubbed by their antagonists " pigeons " because of the number of those birds frequenting their buildings, and the latter " pigs " because their saint, as it was alleged, was always followed by a pig. Whatever truth there may be in the legend (probably none), the association of that useful beast with the hospital is a fact. Stowe says that in his youth, whenever the overseers of the city markets found a pig in bad condition and unfit for human food they slit it in the ear and handed it over to the hospital proctors, who placed a bell round its neck and turned it on to the streets, there to feed on the " Dunguehills." No one appropriated the animals, but many fed them, so that they would follow their benefactors whining, and when waxed fat they became valuable property for the hospital. Stowe states that the actual site of the school was in Bartholomew Lane (east of the present Bank of England), " and so uppe to Three Needle Streete " ; and that of famous men who had been scholars there were Sir Thomas More and our old friend John Whitgift.[1]

St. Giles's Without Cripple Gate.—Tanner calls it a hospital of French order, which would make it an alien house. It was dedicated to St. Giles in the time of Edward I. Though Henry V. dissolved it, there was a refoundation as a fraternity. After its final dissolution, Sir John Gresham, Lord Mayor of London, purchased it for £1,276 10s., Edward VI. granting him a patent. There is no statement in *Monasticon* as to hospital provision.

St. Katharine's By the Tower was founded in 1148 by Maud, queen of Stephen, for the repose of the souls of her son Baldwin and her daughter Matilda, who had both died before her, and for the maintenance of a master, brothers and sisters and several poor persons. In 1273, the prior and brotherhood having purloined the goods and neglected their duties, Eleanor, queen of Henry III., having instituted an action at law, which led to the dissolution of the convent, reconstituted it for a master, three sisters, chaplains, ten bedeswomen, who were to pray for the souls of the foundress, her progenitors and the faithful, and six poor scholar-boys to assist in Divine service.

Here resided for a time, according to *Old and New London*, which does not give its authority for the statement, Raymund Lully (*c.* 1255–1315), in the time of Edward II. This remarkable man had, in the beginning of his career, ecstatic visions, and remained to the end of his long life an enthusiastic preacher, an

---

[1] *Survey of London*, by John Stowe, citizen, 1598, 2nd and extended edition, 1603.

antagonist to the accepted scholastic philosophy, and an ardent advocate of missions and schools, besides being a student of Arabian literature and refuter of Islam, a romance writer and a poet. Lully, if he must be regarded as an eccentric thinker, was certainly a man before his time, and, as a literary artist, worthy of high esteem.[1]

Queen Phillipa, the noble wife of Edward III., attached a chantry at St. Katharine's and increased the endowments of the hospital, besides contributing to the rebuilding of the church, about 1340.

Thomas de Beckington, master in 1435, obtained from Henry VI. an annual Fair lasting three weeks. He was afterwards Bishop of Bath and Wells, and is thought by Ducarel to have rebuilt the nave. An avaricious later master sold the hospital rights in the fair.

Henry VIII. and Katharine of Aragon engrafted upon the foundation the Guild of St. Barbara in 1518, to which many of the highest nobility belonged. As a valuation was taken in 26th Henry VIII., just before the great Dissolution, it is inferred that he intended its destruction, but he had recently married Anne Boleyne and perhaps her intercession saved it. However this may be, saved it was, and continued till the making of the docks necessitated the removal of this seven-hundred-year-old institution. To judge from Walter Besant's *The World went very well then*, people

[1] Dr. FitzMaurice Kelly writes on Raymund Lully in the *Encyc. Brit.*, and Havelock Ellis in the *Contemporary Review* for 1906. In *Old and New London* it is stated that Edward II. employed him at the Tower to transmute baser metals into gold, but Havelock Ellis says that Lully, though he studied alchemy *inter alia*, had no belief in transmutation. The alchemists were the precursors of modern chemistry, and were by no means wholly occupied with transmutation.

[I have seen somewhere quite recently some reference to a translation of Lully's or Lull's work.—J.M.H.]

in latter days lived at St. Katharine's who could not be classed either as poor bedeswomen or poor bedesmen. It survives in spirit as the headquarters of the Queen's Nurses in Regent's Park.

There are two seals of St. Katharine's extant. One simply displays the figure of the patron saint. The other is evidently of Elizabeth's time, for she gave a new charter and the seal bears the arms of England and France crowned and supported by the lion and dragon, and has the legend which reads, anglicised : Seal of the Queen's majesty for the cause of the Church.

St. Mary Spital, Bishopsgate Without.—A Priory of canons and a hospital for poor brothers, all of the order of St. Augustine, was founded by Walter Brune, Roesia his wife, and others, Walter Fitz Eilred giving the site, in 1197. In 1235, it was refounded and styled " The New Hospital of our Lady." At the Dissolution, it is said, it had *180 beds for the reception of sick persons and travellers.* Henry VIII. granted it to John Hales, through whom it passed to the Vaughan family. A pulpit cross stood in the forecourt, but nothing remained in 1830 save part of a stone doorway with a " staple for the hanging of a postern door." Walter Brune and his wife were buried before the altar of the church.

Charing Cross.—In the time of Henry III., William, or Walter, Mareschall, Earl of Pembroke, gave several tenements in Charing to the prior of Rosida Valle in Navarre and a hospital or chapel was erected as chief cell in England on the site. Leland says it was suppressed as an alien house by the act of Henry V., but restored for a fraternity by Edward IV. In the time of Henry VIII., we read of a master, brethren and sisters

and, though nothing is said of poor inmates, the title
of " Hospital of St. Mary Rouncevall " suggests that
provision was made for such. It was granted by
Edward VI. to Sir Thomas Carwardine, Master of the
King's Revels, and associated with Bletchingley Place
in Surrey, the residence of Queen Anne of Cleves.
Northumberland House was erected on the site of this
hospital.[1]

Elsing's Hospital, near Cripplegate, was founded in
1330 by William Elsing for *a hundred blind men*, and
lasted till the Dissolution.

It may be supposed that everyone has been told in
his childhood the legend of Dick Whittington and his
Cat, a story proved by C. L. Kingsford, the historian,
to be apocryphal. It seems to have originated in
adaptation of a folk-lore tale, common on the continent
in the thirteenth century and later, traced as far as
Persia, to a play written in 1605. There is actually a
stone set up in Holloway Road commemorating this
myth by its presence, but only bearing the dates of his
offices. That Richard Whittington became a city
magnate of great wealth is true, but he belonged to an
old Gloucestershire family, and his father was a knight.
He thus started on his career under favourable circumstances. Dying a widower and childless, he left
all his vast wealth for charitable purposes, over and
above what he did in his lifetime. After rebuilding St.
Michael Royal Church, Paternoster, he founded by
will a College associated with an almshouse for thirteen
poor people, the chief of which was called Tutor. This
was in 1424. The College did not survive the Dissolu-

[1] *Monasticon.*

tion, but the Almshouse remains to this day, not indeed in the City but at Highgate, where it is maintained by the Mercers' Company, with which Whittington was closely associated. The editors of *Monasticon* state that in their time (1830) the men had coats and breeches every third year, and the women gowns and petticoats.

St. Bartholomew's, Smithfield.—Rahere, a man born of low degree, became court minstrel (some say jester) to Henry Beauclerc, youngest son of the Conqueror. The story goes that while ill in Rome he vowed to St. Bartholomew, who appeared to him, that if he recovered he would build a hospital " in recreation of poor men." Rahere became an ecclesiastic and, obtaining a site at Smithfield in London from King Henry I., he began there the building of a priory and hospital, the former being placed by him under Augustinian canons, while each had a separate organisation and seals. This was about 1123, and, while Rahere was employed in building, his friend, Alfane, set himself to " compass and go about the high places [? ways] of the church busily to seek and provide necessaries to the need of the poor men that lay in the hospital," and he won over the butchers of Smithfield to contribute. From this it is evident that Smithfield was already a centre of the meat trade. In the book of foundation we may read—" Who should not be astonished there to see, constructed and builded, the honourable building of Pity ? " There were three chapels—possibly terminations of the infirmary—besides the churches known as St. Bartholomew the Great and St. Bartholomew the Less. Diverse sick were placed in the hospital, including *even the insane*, but not, apparently, lepers. Ten years later, Bartholomew

Fair, on St. Bartholomew's Day, was inaugurated by
charter of Henry I. for the benefit of the hospital,
lasted a fortnight for several centuries, and was only
discontinued in 1855. Rahere's beautiful altar tomb
still exists in the church of St. Bartholomew the Great,
as we see in *Fig.* 35.

St. Bartholomew's weathered the storm at the
Dissolution, through the public spirit and energy of the
citizens of London, headed by Lord Mayor Gresham.
They petitioned Henry VIII. on behalf of it and of St.
Mary's Bethlehem, and St. Thomas' in Southwark,
stating that these institutions were " for aid and comfort of the poor, sick, blind, aged and impotent persons,
being not able to help themselves nor having any place
certain where they may be lodged." The petitioners,
moreover, promised that if the King would grant the
governance to them, these places should be reformed—
evidently there had been abuses—and their usefulness
increased so that " greater number . . . shall be
refreshed . . . healed and cured of their infirmities,
frankly and freely, by physicians, surgeons and apothe-
caries, so that all impotent persons not able to labour
shall be relieved . . . and all sturdy beggars not willing
to labour shall be punished, so that . . . few or no persons
shall be seen abroad to beg or ask for alms."[1] We may
notice, even here, mixed motives, not wholly of pity.
Six years later, in 1544, St. Bartholomew's, having in
the meantime become " vacant and altogether destitute
of a master and all fellows and brethren," the king
magnanimously granted the petition of the citizens,
giving to the hospital the title of " The House of the

[1] R. M. Clay, *op. cit.*

PLATE XIX.

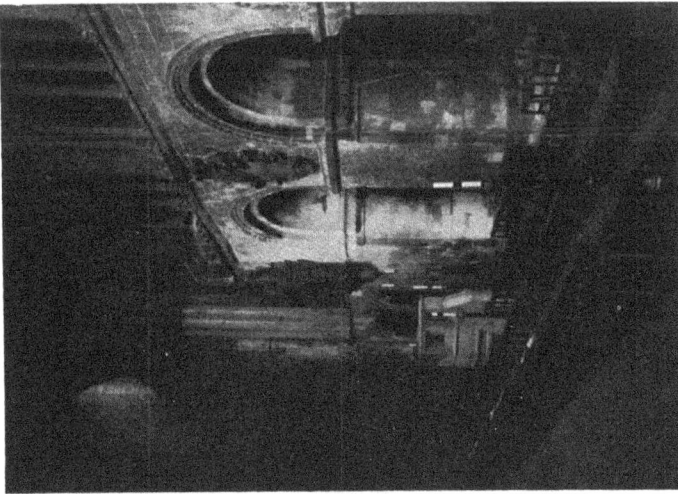

Fig. 34.—ST. BARTHOLOMEW THE GREAT

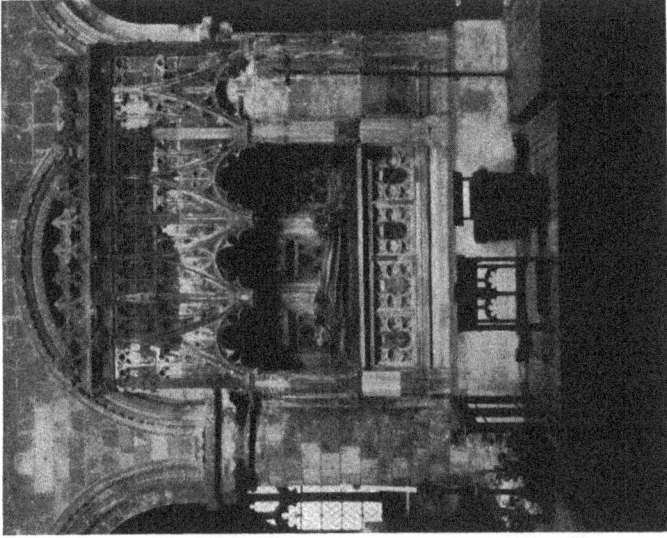

Fig. 35.—RAHERE'S TOMB

[*Face p. 160*

Poor in West Smithfield of the Foundation of King Henry VIII." He endowed it (from possessions then vested in the Crown) with 500 marks yearly, the citizens providing an equal sum, besides nearly £1,000 for refitting it for one hundred patients and necessary supplies. In 1552 there was a design for further increasing its benefits, it being stated that the time was one " when the misery of the poor most seemeth to awake."

St. Mary's of the Star of Bethlehem, above mentioned in the petition of the citizens, was also rescued. Founded originally in 1247 at Bishopsgate Without by Simon Fitzmary, it was specially intended for the housing of the Bishop and Canons of the Mother Church on the Continent on their visitations to England. It was mentioned as a hospital in 1330, but the earliest record of lunatics being received into it was in 1403. St. Mary's was handed over to the City of London by Henry VIII., with all its revenues, afterwards removed to Moorfields, and finally to its present site at Lambeth. The Royal Bethlehem Hospital, as it is now styled, is one of the oldest foundations for the detention of lunatics in Europe.

The ideas regarding insanity in the Middle Ages, and long after, did not admit of its treatment as a physical disease, although, as we have seen, mad people were taken in St. Bartholomew's.[1] There, as elsewhere, the miraculous was sought and credited with cure. Men did not realise then, as they have hardly done at the present day, the vast and perennial miracle of " Vis

---

[1] *Monasticon* records the existence of a hospital at Chester before *temp.* Henry III. for poor and " silly " people. See also pp. 39 and 40.

medicatrix Naturæ," the healing power of Nature, without which the wisest physician, the most skilful surgeon, or the astutest alienist can accomplish nothing. The belief that lunatics (moon-struck) were possessed of devils or influenced by witchcraft or some other occult agencies is very old.   We see that the Jews, in the time of Jesus, held that view.   The demons had to be driven forth by exorcism or other means.   Flagellation was one of these, and Miss Clay describes a thirteenth century window at Canterbury in which is depicted a maniac tied with ropes and dragged by his friends to the shrine of St. Thomas, while they belabour him on the way.   In another part of the same window the man is represented free and returning thanks for his recovery.

Flagellation as a form of religious exercise is traceable to antiquity : it was practised among the Egyptians, Jews, Greeks and Romans.   At the Roman Lupercalia,[1] women were flogged to avert sterility or as a purificatory ceremony.   As early as the eleventh century the Church recognised flagellation as a form of penance.   Flagellants appeared in northern Italy in 1260 and spread to Central Europe, but never, it would seem, to this country.   Although considered a heresy by the highest dignatories of the Church, this phase of fanaticism was never wholly repressed as a popular form of religious zeal, but, with various recrudescences, continued into the nineteenth century and is even to be witnessed in a modified form among Latin races at the present day.[2] It seems, therefore, a fair inference that castigation of the insane had its origin in some notion of *beating out*

---

[1] A trace of this practice is seen in *Julius Cæsar*, Act I., Sc. II.
[2] *Encyc. Brit.*, " Flagellants," by Prof. P. A. Alphandéry.

the evil influence, and that the " conservativeness of ancient habit " was the cause of its being maintained till comparatively modern times.   Indeed, the fettering and beating of mad people so long prevailed in England that " Bedlam " has become a byword for a confusion of loud voices, such as issued from Bethlehem and other places where the insane were incarcerated and shamefully treated.

It is a relief to turn from these benighted notions and their outcome to more enlightened ideas and methods in other lands.   The ancient Egyptians and Greeks followed a sympathetic method which included music, the appeal of the beautiful in Nature and in Art, and employment without unnecessary restraint.   What was the treatment in the asylum at Bagdad, mentioned on p. 5, is unknown to the present writer, but from what we know of the Arabs in the early years of the Caliphate, with their freedom from much of the superstition which hampered their Christian contemporaries, we may surmise that it was more rational than that generally obtaining in Europe.   Yet close to our own shores, to wit, at Gheel in Belgium, the shrine of St. Dymphna was famed so early as the seventh century for its miraculous power of healing.   Hither were brought the mentally afflicted from all over Europe, till by the seventeenth it had grown to be " a unique colony for the insane."   It and the adjacent farming hamlets " provide at the present day homes, board and care for nearly 2,000 insane persons under medical and government supervision."[1]

[1] Dr. Frederick Peterson, in *Encyc. Brit.*, 1911, " Insanity, hospital treatment."

Merchant Taylors' Hospital.—The Merchant Taylors were originally a Guild of " Linen Armourers " which received its first licence from Edward I. They were really merchants as well as artificers. " Their first master, Henry de Ryall, was called their ' pilgrim,' as one who travelled for the whole company, and their wardens ' purveyors of dress.' " They made, besides men's and women's raiment, quilted surcoats for soldiers, the padded lining for armour, and probably the trappings for war-horses, etc., hence their original title. Edward III. granted them letters patent, and became a member of their company. These privileges were confirmed by successive sovereigns, and Henry VII., who also joined the fraternity, changed their name to " Merchant Taylors." Their silver yard was their standard of measurement and used at Bartholomew's Fair and elsewhere. Whether or no Threadneedle Street (Three Needle, as Stowe says) took its name from them, their fourteenth-century home was there. This was called the New Hall or Taylors' Inn, in succession to a still more ancient place in Basing Lane, Cheapside. Goodman's drawing of 1599, reproduced in Wilkinson's *Londinia Illustrata* shows Taylors' Inn and Hospital of that date, with the three gables of the latter in the middle. The almshouses were later removed to Rosemary Street, and provided homes for widows of the Company. It would seem, however, that men were admitted to the original hospital, for it is recorded that John Churchman, a past master of the Company, was allowed in 1610 " to wear his bedesman's gown without a badge " and was not required " to appear in the hall with the other pensioners." Hence it seems a fair

PLATE XX.

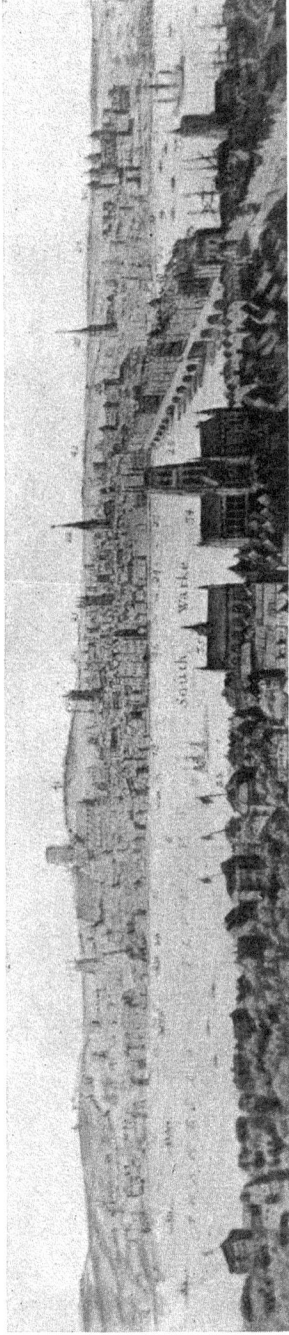

Fig. 36.—LONDON BEFORE THE GREAT FIRE
Wilkinson's Londinia Illustrata

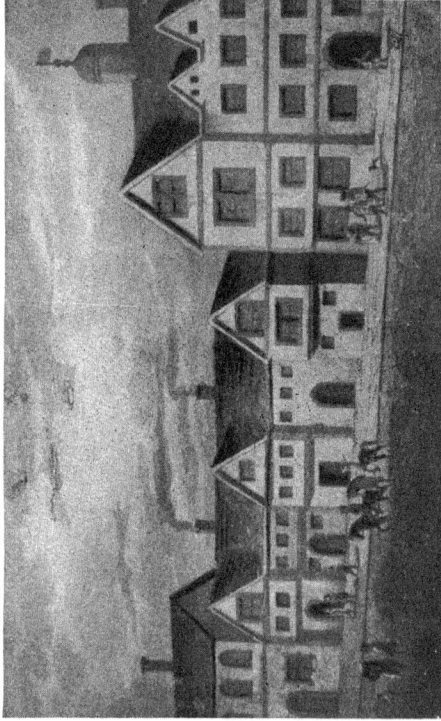

Fig. 37.—MERCHANT TAYLORS'
Londinia Illustrata

[Face p. 164

inference that the hospital was never intended for any but members of the society, or those connected with it.

The Merchant Taylors' School was founded in 1561, by Richard Hills, who was Master of the Company in 1599, and afterwards transferred to new buildings on the site of Sutton's School at Charter House from its original situation in St. Lawrence Pountney. In anticipation of this, Sir Thomas White, another member, founded St. John's College, Oxford, and reserved forty-three out of fifty endowed scholarships for boys from the school. The number was at first 250, now it is 520. The object of the foundation was stated to be " for the better education and bringing up of children in good manners and literature." The school is entirely supported by the Company. Taylors' Hall was destroyed in the Fire of London, when, it is stated, " the Company's plate was melted into a lump of two hundred pounds." The present Hall is on the same site in Threadneedle Street, where it was rebuilt in 1671.[1]

The Great Palace of the Savoy should be included amongst the London hospitals, though its service in that character was brief. This pile of buildings, fronting the river a little to the west of Somerset House, is figured by Miss Clay and in *Old and New London*. First built by Simon de Montfort in 1245, it acquired its name from being granted by Henry III. to Peter

---

[1] *Encyc. Brit.*, " Livery Companies."
Old and New London.
City Companies of London, by P. H. Ditchfield, 1904.
[I am informed by the Clerk of the Merchant Taylors' Company that " the school is not, and never has been, limited to the children of the Company or its servants."—J. M. H.]

M

of Savoy, uncle to his queen Eleanor of Provence. The Queen gave it to her second son, Edmund, Earl of Lancaster, and it long remained part of the Duchy of Lancaster. The French king, John, lived here a captive after the Battle of Poictiers, and here he died after his voluntary return. During the peasants' revolt of 1381, the Savoy suffered much damage through the unpopularity of John of Gaunt, Shakespeare's " time-honoured Lancaster " in *King Richard II*. It was beautifully restored by Henry VII. in 1509 as a hospital for 100 poor people. Edward VI.'s commissioners could find no irregularities ; nevertheless, it was dissolved and, though Queen Mary restored its functions as a hospital, the intentions of its founders were not long thereafter fulfilled. All that remains of this once " fairest manor in England " is the hospital chapel restored by Sydney Smirk, the architect, at the cost of Queen Victoria, and known as the Chapel Royal Savoy. The ancient frontage to the Thames is covered by the Victoria Embankment.

Charter House.—St. Bruno was the founder of the Carthusian order. Samuel Herne, who had been a Carthusian scholar, recounts a legend in his *Domus Carthusiana*, 1677. Bruno was in the act of burying a greatly-esteemed friend when the dead man rose on his bier and declared himself condemned to eternal punishment for his sins. " If this good man," thought he, " is thus committed to Hell-fire, how shall I, who have come so short of his merit, escape ? " Thereupon he called to him six companions, and agreed with them to live thenceforth a life wholly devoted to religion. These seven came to the Bishop of Grenoble and explained to him their wishes. Pursuant to this, they built for themselves three huts and an oratory on a desolate spot known as Chartreuse, among the mountains above the rivers Isère and Drac in south-eastern France, rocky and snow-covered throughout a great part of the year, and gave themselves up to a life of prayer, silence and extreme austerity. This was in 1084. They wore the coarsest garments, ate sparingly, spent the time, each in his separate little house, save for cultivating their limited grounds, assembling in church for the major offices and in the refectory on feast days only. There has never been any very great extension of Carthusian priories, and no essential modification of the rule. At the Dissolution, there were nine priories in England, the most important being at Sheen in Surrey and Smithfield, where Charter House is a corruption of Chartreuse.

It is curious to observe a certain " irony of fate " in later inversions of the Carthusian tradition. At St. Cross, Beaufort, who was never a Carthusian, planned self-contained dwellings for the brethren and gave them a banqueting hall, while, much later, Sutton provided for men who dine daily in the refectory or guest house of the long departed Carthusians.

In the time of Edward III. a terrible plague, the Black Death, ravaged Europe and spread from the western counties of England to London. So many people died in the city that a Bishop of London bought a plot of land, called " No man's land," in Smithfield for a place of burial, and Sir Walter de Manny, a Netherlander, and created a knight of the Garter by Edward III. for military services to him, acquired a contiguous piece of land from the priory of St. Bartholomew in 1349 for the same purpose, building there a chapel for the souls of the departed. It would appear that de Manny and Michael de Northburgh, a later Bishop of London, were both concerned in the foundation on this spot of a Carthusian priory known as " La Salutation Mère Dieu," a bull of Pope Urban V. referring to this priory in 1362. There is some obscurity on this point, but it is certain that de Manny did obtain Letters patent from Edward III., authorising or confirming his establishment, in 1371.

At the Dissolution, the prior, John Houghton and four monks were hung for refusing to take the oath of supremacy, eight others died in prison, and a mutilated portion of the prior's body was suspended from the gate as a warning to the rest. Contemporary writers comment adversely on the obstinacy and contumacy of these men, and praise the succeeding prior for his acquiescence in the surrender. After passing through the hands of one or two owners, the place was acquired by the Howard family for some £2,000, who made a palace of it, and finally it was sold by the Earl of Suffolk, son of the Duke of Norfolk, to Sir Thomas Sutton for £13,000.

Sutton (c. 1532–1611) does not seem to have been of high birth, but was a man of education and acquired vast wealth, particularly from coalfields in the county of Durham. The motto to his arms (probably granted) is *Deo Dante Dedi*, to God, the giver, I have given, and is eloquent of his motives. He had previously obtained an Act of Parliament authorising him to establish a hospital and free school at Hallingbury Bouchers, in

Essex, but, finding Smithfield more suitable, he was granted letters patent from James I. to place them there.   The foundation consisted of a corporation of governors chosen from men of high station with power to add to their number as vacancies occurred, who had complete control.   The provision was for eighty pensioners who were, variously, gentlemen by descent but fallen into poverty (such as Colonel Newcome of Thackeray's *The Newcomes*), soldiers who had borne arms by sea or land, servants of the King's household, or merchants decayed by piracy or shipwreck.   Their ages were not to be under 50 years unless they had been disabled in actual warfare, when they might be admitted at 40.   A school was attached for 44 poor boys with a master and usher to teach reading, writing, grammar, Latin and Greek.   Sutton gave ample endowments from his numerous estates, provided £8,000 for building of hospital, chapel and school, £1,090 as a beginning of stock, and £26 3s. 4d. in trust for each of his "feoffees."   The beneficiaries were to have clothing, food, lodging and " wages," and there was power to extend if revenue increased.   Over all was the Master, who was also to be preacher.   The brethren were not permitted to bring their wives, if they had any, neither must they interfere with the business of the hospital ; they had to attend at the chapel and must not frequent taverns, especially *when attired in their gowns*.   The style of the place was to be " The Governors and Hospital of King James."   At least, that was their official designation, but we may be sure, from the title given by Herne's book, published only some fifty years later, that the name had been from first

" Charter House," and the inmates popularly called
" Carthusians."[1]

Thackeray, who became a Carthusian when a fatherless boy of eleven, refers frequently to his old school in
his works, first as " Slaughter House " and " Smithfield," but later, in mellowed retrospect, as " Grey
Friars." His allusions to Charter House and its inmates,
in *The Newcomes*, are short, but reveal an intimate
knowledge. What he says about Colonel Newcome, the
old gentleman who was bent on answering " adsum "
at roll-call, in this connection, is tender and pathetic,
and the "red-cheeked " little gown-boy, the old man's
friend, might have been himself.

Christ's Hospital was founded by the young Edward
VI., who has also to his credit other schools with charitable intent, such as the free grammar school in Birming-
ham, of which the author has lively memory of morning
thanksgiving for " our pious founder, King Edward
the Sixth." The celebrated " Bluecoat School " was
established upon the site of the dissolved Priory of
the Franciscans or Grey Friars in Newgate Street and
not far from Charter House. The Grey Friars' house
was repaired in 1552 and nearly 400 fatherless children
were admitted. It is recorded that on Christmas Day,
the same year, the scholars lined the adjacent streets
to the number of 340, " all in one livery of russet cotton
. . . And the Easter after they were in blue at the
Spittle, and so have continued ever since." Senior
readers may remember, like the author, the Bluecoat
boys kicking about footballs in the forecourt during

---

[1] *Monasticon.*
  Domus Carthusiana, Samuel Herne, scholar at Charter House and fellow
of Clare Hall, Cambridge, 1677.

Plate XXI.

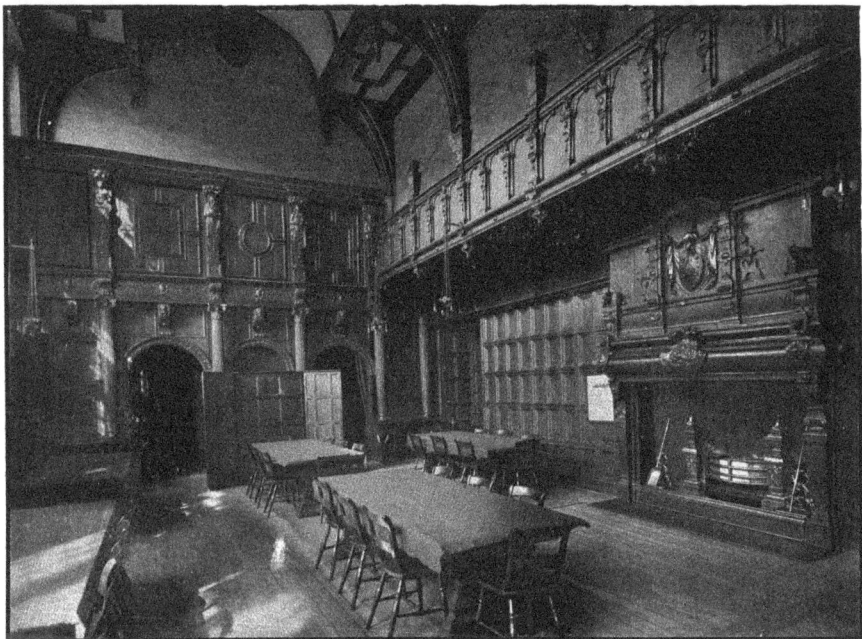

Fig. 38.—CHARTER HOUSE, BANQUETING HALL

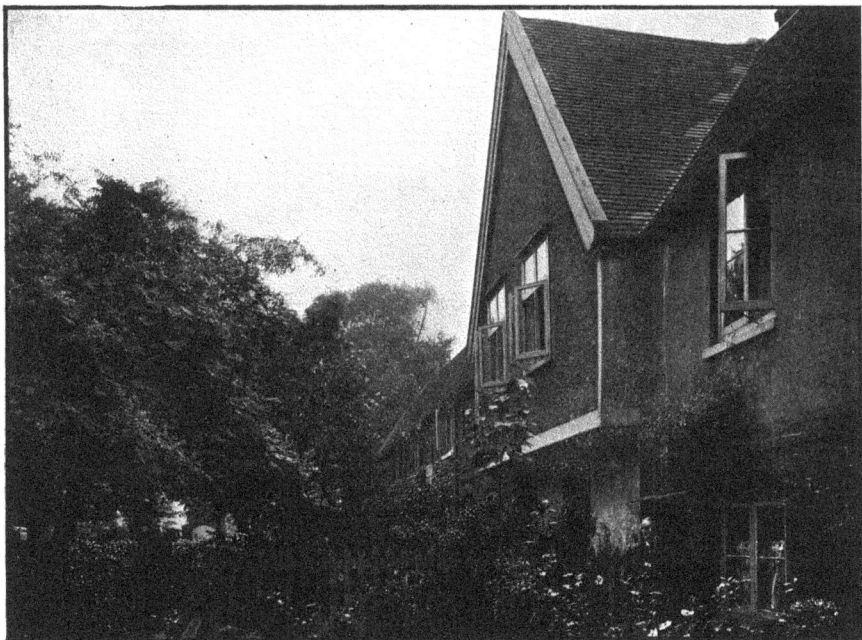

Fig 39.—MONOUX'S ALMSHOUSES, WALTHAMSTOW

Both prints by permission of the Underground Co.

[*Face p. 170*

recess with the skirts of their long coats tucked through their belts, in the days before they were translated to Horsham in Sussex.   Their cumbrous and antiquated uniform is *minus* hat or cap, not, it has been stated, because it does not exist in theory, but is too small for wearing.[1]

[1] *Cf.* p. 22 and Fig. 2 respecting Chetham's Hospital, Manchester.

CHAPTER XV

LONDON SOUTH OF THE RIVER

Southwark and Bermondsey lie in that part of Surrey bounded by the Thames as it flows between Vauxhall and Deptford. Long before the Claudian invasion in A.D. 43, the lower reaches of the river were subject to tidal flooding, and the Romans, with the engineering skill for which they were famous, built a continuous embankment along the shore in the area we are considering. This enabled them to make it habitable, and to erect upon it the villas whose vestiges we trace in those tessellated pavements discovered far below the present surface. Neglect of the Roman works probably enabled the Anglo-Saxon invaders to row their ships above London Bridge, and Canute to do much the same thing later, by way of the tidal marshes which had resumed their sway. Right through the Middle Ages, the maintenance of the embankments caused endless trouble, and the present level, covered with houses and intersecting streets, several feet below high-water, is only kept dry by artificial means. Indeed, this part might not inaptly be called a little Holland in London.[1]

Southwark and Bermondsey are hardly separable, either historically or topographically. Southwark derives its names from affording the southern defences of London in Anglo-Saxon days, while its early incorpora-

---

[1] *Surrey Archæol Colls.,* Vol. XXVIII. Codrington, London, S. of the Thames.

tion gave it the title of " The Borough," which has ever since clung to it. There were from early times, *Three Principal Parishes* in the district, namely, St. Margaret's in Southwark, St. Olif's, and St. Mary Magdalene's in Bermondsey. We will first consider St. Olif's, better known as St. Olave's through a corruption. Olaf is still a favourite name in Norway, and is borne by the Crown Prince, son of our own Maud, sister of King George. When Olaf Trygvason, the famous king, came to spread Christianity in Norway, Olaf Haraldson was a boy and was baptised. On the death of Trygvason in battle, the kingdom passed under the sway of Sweyn, King of Denmark, whereupon young Olaf, cut off from his kingdom, became a viking (pirate) under the age of twelve. In 1014 Sweyn had overrun England with his Danes, and Ethelred the Unready had fled to France. On the sudden death of Sweyn, Ethelred returned to his kingdom and invited those who would join him and take his pay to help him in driving out the Danes. Olaf was one of these, and brought to the King's aid a great troop of northmen. They sailed up the Thames, and are said to have brought about the fall of London Bridge by chaining their boats to its piers and rowing hard down stream. However this may be, the Danes were driven from their strongholds at the Tower and in Southwark. Olaf fought further successful battles against them in Kent and East Anglia, and was rewarded by Ethelred with leave to collect £21,000, or even more, according to some, from the people of the land. Returning at length to his native land, Olaf endeavoured to spread Christianity among his people, with extreme severity, and eventually fell fighting against his enemies and some of his own subjects whom he had alienated by his high-handedness. Nevertheless, he became canonised by the people of Norway[1] and the patron saint, not only of the church we are considering but of three others in London, namely, Hart Street in the City, one of the few ancient City churches which survived the Great Fire[2], where Pepys, the diarist, attended, and where his monument was later erected; Hanbury Street in Stepney; and Woodbury Down, Finsbury.[3] " Tooley " is a further corruption of " Olaf," and is well known as the name of a street on the old level behind London Bridge Stations. It is interesting and amusing to refer to some wills in connection with this parish. These are quoted in Vol. I of the Surrey Archæological Collections, 1854, in which year, and in the Borough of Southwark, that Society was inaugurated.

Will of John Burchestre, knight, 1466—" My body to be buried in the wall beside the Holy King St. Olave in Southwark." Sir John's " Holy King " was evidently otherwise armed and his effigy appears to have been removed and restored to its place some 90 years after, for we read in the churchwardens' accounts of 1556–8 these entries—" Item paid to John Carowe for making a scepter and an axe for St. Towle iijs, iiijd "; then later, " Item paid to Modyn for St. Olaf xxxs. Item pd. more for a dinner when we set him up ijs viijd." Further

[1] Baring Gould's *Lives of the Saints*.
[2] Sir L. Gomme's *The Making of London*.
[3] It would seem from this, though the people in the country generally deemed Olaf's " collection " little less obnoxious than the Danes' incursions, that the inhabitants of London cherished a lively gratitude to him. Baring Gould observes that the term " saint " must be stretched to its utmost in order to include Olaf in the meaning of it. He gives a representation of Olaf seated and with a great two-edged sword. *Cf.* Churchwardens' accounts.

in the will appears—" Item I will that an honest priest be found for to sing at the altar of St. John in the said church of St. Olave by x years next following after my decease for my soul," etc.   John Alynson, 1543, wills to be buried in the "Church of Saynte Owlyf," and Henry Leeke, 1563, in "St. Olyve's."   This last spelling suggests a pacivity far removed from the character of the " Holy King."   There appears no record of a hospital in St. Olave's parish, but a school as established in Queen Elizabeth's time, as we shall see on p. 180.

The Municipal Borough of Bermondsey occupies the right bank of the Thames between London Bridge and Limehouse Reach, and includes the Surrey Commercial Docks and Rotherhithe, long associated with shipping and largely figuring in Walter Besant's *The World went very well then*.   The first part of the name is probably patronymic, and the second, meaning an island, is common to it and several other places on both sides of the river, such as Battersea, Putney, Chelsea, Molesey, and Thorney, the site of Westminster Abbey.

Bermondsey Abbey.—Aldwin Child, a citizen of London, began a church about 1082 to the honour of the Holy Saviour and St. Mary Magdalene for monks from the Cluniac Priory of La Charité sur Loire, and it is mentioned in Domesday as a fair church newly built. This was augmented by William II. with the royal demesne in Bermondsey and other revenues.   There had been a Norman palace in the same parish, perhaps succeeding a pre-Conquest one, like that in Kennington where Hardicanute is said to have died.   Henry I. gave this Bermondsey house to the priory to enlarge it. After a long succession of foreign priors, Richard Denton, an

Englishman, became the Superior, and he obtained in Richard Il.'s reign the denization of the house, thus saving it from suppression when, later, alien cells were so treated. Denton resigned in 1391, and in 1399, at Richard II.'s request, John Attilburgh was created first abbot by Pope Boniface IX., the Priory being thus elevated to the dignity of an Abbey. The last abbot was Robert Wharton, who was created Bishop of St. Asaph in 1536, having previously obtained a dispensation to hold the Abbey *in commendam*. Being so far nicely provided for, he surrendered the Abbey to Henry in the following year, receiving a pension of 500 marks, equal to £333 6s. 8d. The property eventually came into the hands of Sir Thomas Pope, who is said to have destroyed the church and other buildings to make himself a house with the materials. The gate-house, the last remaining fragment, was removed in 1805. This is one among many other evidences of the indifference to the beautiful in architecture of that age and of our forefathers', almost down to our own time.[1]

Southwark Cathedral.—There is another church over against St. Olave's, but on the other side of the bridge-foot. This was at first called St. Mary's Overy, belonging to an Augustinian Priory till the Dissolution, after which it was named St. Saviour's and in 1904 created Southwark Cathedral. It is a beautiful example of the Early English style, though there are slight remains of the earlier Norman fabric. In the north nave aisle is a fine monument of the poet Gower, a friend of Geoffrey Chaucer. The bishops of Winchester

[1] *Encyc. Brit.*, " Bermondsey." *Monasticon.* Memorials of Old Surrey, edited by Rev. J. C. Cox, 1911.

had a town house on Bankside, skirting the river, and the arms of Cardinal Beaufort are displayed in the south transept.

The origin of St. Mary's Overy Priory is uncertain, but we are on firm ground when we read of the foundation being renewed in 1106 for Augustinian canons regular by two knights, William Pont d'Arch and William Dauncey, and of William Giffard, Bishop of Winchester, building the nave of the church in 1107. Giffard has left his name in history as the friend of the much more celebrated Archbishop Anselm, as aiding the first Cistercian settlement in England and as restoring his Cathedral with great magnificence.

Origin of St. Thomas'.—Just a hundred years after the foundation of St. Mary's Overy, to wit, in 1207, there was a terrible fire in which the greater part of Southwark was consumed, and the Priory perished. Thereupon the monks built a temporary house, near their own, which they called a Hospital, while their old home was being rebuilt. In 1213 Thomas, Prior of Bermondsey, founded a hospital adjoining the wall of his own monastery for converts from Judaism and poor children. Peter de Rupibus, Bishop of Winchester, whose munificence caused the rebuilding of St. Mary's in Southwark, in the beautiful manner we have noticed, disliked the site of its hospital and caused it to be removed to the other side of the road through the borough on to land belonging to Amicius, archdeacon of Surrey, who became its first custos or Warden, and dedicated to St. Thomas the Martyr. But Bishop Peter, deeming the hospital in Bermondsey too restricted in scope, caused the two hospitals to be united in one foundation under canons regular, yet free from control of St. Mary's Overy. To this the brethren and sisters of Bermondsey hospital were transferred in 1215.

The first prior of St. Mary's Overy was Algod, 1106, and the last, Bartholomew Linsted, who surrendered the priory on October 14th, 1539, receiving a pension of £100 a year.

The further history of St. Thomas' Hospital is as follows. At the Dissolution, when it fell in spite of the citizens' petition to Henry VIII., it had a Master, brethren and three lay sisters, and provided for *forty* poor, infirm, and impotent folk. The young king, Edward VI., has the credit of refounding it as a house for the cure of the sick, and as such it has ever since remained. St. Thomas', having been granted by the King to the Mayor and Citizens of London, was repaired by them in 1552, for during the interval after Dissolution it had fallen into much decay. In 1558 it was incorporated by charter, and was styled for a time " The King's Hospital in Southwark."[1] The earlier buildings were replaced by others in 1702, but these are now represented by offices and the chapter house of Southwark Cathedral. *Old and New London* gives an illustration of the hospital in 1840, which shows a statue of the king in the forecourt.

St. Thomas' much younger but equally famous sister, founded by Thomas Guy in 1721, on the opposite side of St. Thomas' Street, gave rise by its presence to

---

[1] The common seal of St. Mary's Overy is described in *Monasticon* as showing a figure of the Virgin and Child surrounded by a scroll with the words—Ave. Maria. Plena. Dominus. Tecum. Benedicta.—and four encircling angels. *Monasticon.* Manning and Bray's *Survey of Surrey.*

a degree of rivalry between their respective students till the elder hospital was removed in 1871 to the present splendid range of buildings opposite the Houses of Parliament.

A Lazar-House was founded some time before 1321 in Kent Street, Southwark, and appears to have been of royal foundation. It was long under the care of St. Bartholomew's Hospital—this may account for lepers not being housed there. The chapel used as a schoolhouse is figured in Wilkinson's *Londinia Illustrata*. See also p. 13.

SCHOOLS. St. Saviour's.—It is not altogether inappropriate to take some notice of early free schools set up in South London, which were, indeed, in their own particular sense, houses of pity. By charter of Elizabeth in 1562, and later by her letters patent, a free school was erected in Southwark. The " high master " had to be " a man holy in body, honest, virtuous, and learned in good clean Latin literature and also in Greek, if any such may be found ; a wedded man, a single man, or a minister that hath no benefice with cure nor service that may let [hinder] his doing business in school." The scholars were limited to a hundred. The statutes were enlarged in 1614 and subscribed by the Bishop of Winchester. The master and usher were enjoined to " wisely mix severity with lenity . . . ever proposing by precept and example to clear up and put life and spirit into the capacity, memory, love, patience, diligence, gentleness and moderate desire in the scholars and prevent all means that may make them dull, forgetful, weary, impatient, negligent, stubborn, and careless of the good report, or have cause to speak ill of the school or forsake it."[1]

Rules for exercise and recreation excluded playing for money or betting, but encouraged chess, use of the long bow, running, leaping, and wrestling. There were scholarships at Oxford and Cambridge.

St. Olave's School.—Elizabeth granted letters patent in 1571, which were confirmed in 1675 by Charles II. The present school is in Tooley Street, after several removals. Part of the endowments came from the neighbouring Horsley Down, which, in 1579, consisted of sixteen acres of grazing land.

In Camberwell a school was founded in 1615, under letters patent of James I., by Rev. Edward Wilson, M.A. The master was to be " a man of wise, sociable and loving disposition, not hasty and furious nor of evil example ; such a one as can discern the nature and disposition of every child ; if such a one can be gotten." He was not to practise physic without the consent of the governors. Only twelve poor parishioners were to be free, besides the sons of the oldest wardens during their last year of office, and the rest had to pay five shillings a quarter and three pence for brooms and rods and a pound of good candles, the week after Michaelmas. The recreations were the same as at St. Saviour's aforesaid.[2]

Southwark Inns.—In Vol. II. of the Surrey Archæological Collections, G. R. Corner, F.S.A., had some notes on Old Inns in Southwark.

---

[1] In Sir L. Gomme's *London*, p. 199, a map of *c.* 1542 is reproduced. The original lettering is mediæval, but, in modern script, " the grammar school, 1562," is marked. St. Margaret's parish church is also shown at some distance from St. Saviour's.

[2] *Jour. Brit. Arch. Association*, Vol. XIV.

The Tabard, immortalised by Chaucer, appears to have originated in 1307 when the Abbot and Convent of Hyde, near Winchester, purchased two houses in Southwark, and the Abbot had licence from the Bishop of Winchester to build a chapel to his Hospitium or guest-house in the parish of St. Margaret in Southwark. At the Dissolution, presumably because it had a chapel, it was granted to John and Thomas Master. The original house was destroyed in the Southwark fire of 1676. Though the name was ignorantly altered to " Talbot " in Aubrey's time, it had been rebuilt, and was standing in 1864. Its memory is retained in Tabard Street. The sixteenth century Tabard is figured in *Old and New London.*

The White Hart was probably founded in the time of Richard II., the sign being one of that king's badges, and is historically associated with the insurrection of 1450, Jack Cade having made his quarters there. It is also the scene of Shakespeare's *King Henry VI.,* part 2. Corner considered that it was rebuilt after the fire in Southwark in 1676 on the ancient model, the open galleries of such inns being commonly used for theatrical purposes. The excellent illustration of this inn as it was in 1864 appeared in the same volume of the Society, and an interesting woodcut in *Old and New London.* The present writer well remembers it in the early " seventies," when he used to take his lunch in a part of the house shown in Corner's picture. The much better known illustration, however, is that in the *Pickwick Papers,* where we are introduced to the immortal Sam Weller cleaning boots of the customers. The White Hart *remains* as it was *to the present moment.*

N

The Site of the Globe Theatre, of which Shakespeare
was joint-owner, and where he acted, has been traced
in Barclay and Perkin's brewery, while the " Bull-
baiting " and the " Bear Garden," shown on old maps
of the district, recall the amusements of the Elizabethan
age and later.

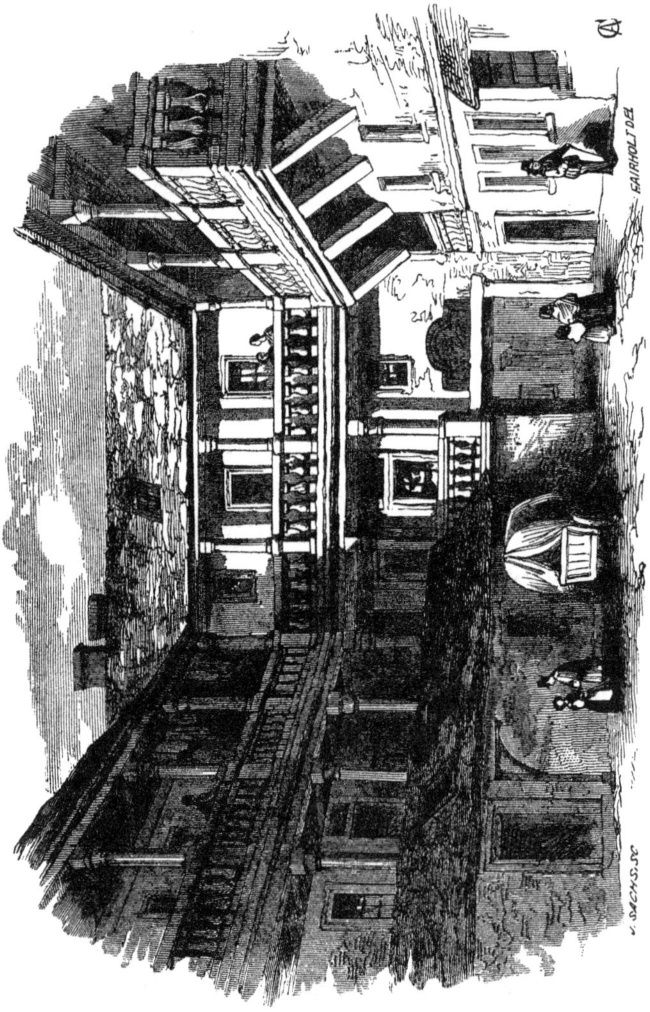

FIG. 40.—THE WHITE HART, SOUTHWARK.
By permission of Surrey Archaeological Society.

CHAPTER XVI

IN looking back over the thousand years that have gone, we see one silver thread passing through them all, round which, like beautiful crystals, have gathered refuges for the poor, the aged, and the infirm. Whatever other motives may have helped to raise these memorials of our fathers' piety, that silver thread of Pity was the unfailing factor.

In surveying the mediæval Houses of Pity, one is struck with the disproportionate attention given by their builders to the chapels. Their great size alone must have absorbed a large proportion of the founders' funds, while their beauty would be above the appreciation of the poor and ignorant pensioners. Yet we must bear in mind three things. Firstly, the chapels were often used for public service as well; secondly, the homes provided were far better than the hovels previously occupied by the inmates; thirdly, and this much the most important, the centuries before the Reformation were eminently religious in a sense distinctive of those early days. The Church was, or claimed to be, paramount in the lives of the people, while the future state was ever present and beset with terrors in the minds of all. These hospital chapels were always works of art, whether in humbler or more aspiring degree, as is attested by still existing examples at St. Cross, St. Mary's Chichester, and Ewelme, as well as by remains and ruins, many of which are figured in Miss Clay's book. Ecclesiastical Art reached unsurpassed attainments in these ages, and was inspired by religious conceptions of which they were, indeed, the highest tangible expression. Men did not know how to build badly, and could not create that which was ugly. In the service of the Divine those old builders felt compelled to give their best. As Emerson sings—

> " The hand that rounded Peter's dome
> And groined the aisles of Christian Rome
> Wrought in a sad sincerity :
> Himself from God he could not free ;
> He builded better than he knew—
> The conscious stone to beauty grew."

We have already observed mixed motives, as typified in the confession of Henry de Blois, and in the preamble of the Duke and Duchess of Suffolk. If in providing for a few only of the poor and stricken at one time (though in the course of years there were many) they were serving themselves, as they believed, by doing a meritorious act and providing for their souls' welfare by many prayers, who can censure them ? Let him whose motives are always pure cast the first stone.

In reading Miss Clay's classic, the fact strikes one that many of the ancient hospitals founded have ceased to be. Out of 800 and more, but comparatively few remain. Although, even at this distance of time, one feels indignant at Henry VIII.'s rapacity and hardness of heart in totally repressing certain hospitals, we must remember that Cromwell's commission preceded each act of dissolution, and that there had been much and widespread abuse, largely through the dishonesty of those entrusted with management. Miss Clay says that this was exceptional, yet the many instances she gives, besides others observed by the present writer, create the impression that corruption did creep in, at one time or another, almost universally.

Where bishops, abbots, or municipalities exercised efficient supervision, abuses could be checked or remedied, but where unrestricted control was left in the hands of wardens or masters or sometimes even of men in higher position, whether lay or clerical, dishonest self-interest would, in the course of centuries, from time to time assert itself. Moreover, even before the Dissolution, untoward circumstances weakened or brought to naught many a house of pity. War and pestilence were among these, as we have seen in the case of St. Leonard's, York. Another adverse condition was the custom of " corridies " by which powerful people, not excepting the sovereign, claimed the right, based generally but not universally on a founder's privileges, to place persons in monasteries and hospitals to be there maintained free. It would take a strong man to resist such demands, though we read of a few so doing, and a continued tax of this nature would obviously weaken the resources of an institution. The decline and disappearance of leprosy would lead to the closing of lazar-houses.

Refoundations.—Of the hospitals which have passed under our survey, the records of 115 furnish enough material for an analysis of the conditions under which they were founded, ceased to be, or survived till modern times. If we give a consideration to the last phase first, we find that a little over one-half come into that category. A few, indeed, were actually dissolved but afterwards refounded, and it will be well to pay attention to these because they form a link between those that perished and those that survived of themselves.

St. John's, Exeter (p. 36), has an interesting history. Its marked ecclesiastical constitution, given by Bishop Grandison, was probably the reason, or *excuse*, for its dissolution by Henry's commissioners. It is not evident that Thomas Carew, to whom the king granted it, was the refounder, though we know that the school, dissolved like many another which had a more or less monastic association, was restored by the Crossing family.

Harnham Hospital, in the city of Salisbury, suffered in like manner, and was restored in 1610 by James I. Wiltshire, be it noted, has the credit of retaining all its ancient hospitals.

Berkshire and Buckingham (Chap. VI.) have four hospitals restored, though the reason why is not manifest. Christ's Hospital, Abingdon, was refounded in the reign of Edward VI. ; Donnington and High Wycombe under Elizabeth ; Newport Pagnell by James I.'s consort, Queen Anne.

King's Lynn (p. 76) survived the storm of Henry's dissolution, but lost its endowments in Edward's time, and did not recover them till the reign of James I. It is probable that the brothers and sisters in this case were simply poor people and not " religious," as in some places. (See pp. 6 & 7.)

We well know the story of St. Thomas', Southwark.

Dissolution.—The supreme interest, however, centres round the question, why were *any* of these Houses of

Pity destroyed rather than why half of them survived. In a valuable article in the *Encyclopædia Britannica* on schools, by Alfred Francis Leach, M.A., he says that grammar schools from quite early times contained an eleemosynary element. For that reason, as has already been remarked in these pages, they should be to that extent numbered among the Houses of Pity. Nevertheless, many schools perished irretrievably at the great Dissolution simply because they had monastic associations. So was it in the case of hospitals. The element of monasticism in their constitution in an age when the Church was the chief bulwark against violence and the only light shining amidst the gross darkness of ignorance became the cause of their undoing in a later age, when a reaction had arisen against what men had come to regard as a kingdom within the kingdom. That separation from the religious supremacy of the Papacy which initiated the Reformation in this country involved the suppression of the monasteries. The two systems could not live side by side, and the weaker had to go under. A detached view, while it cannot exculpate Henry for his violence and greed, must recognise a rising tide against the monasteries. As in all cases of reaction, there was a lack of reasoned judgment, of weighing values one against another. When selfishness and greed are thrown into the scale on the one side, regard for the general welfare and pity on the other " kick the beam." Reasoned judgment and common sense would indicate that the schools and hospitals could all have been re-formed. The monastic element could, at that time, have been beneficially eliminated, the secular and essential purpose retained, and the endowments of the purely conventual establishments used for their enlargement. Yet this was scarcely done. We have seen how a few hospitals were refounded not long after the general Dissolution. A very few (to the writer's knowledge) were reconstituted without dissolution, and a careful study of these cases may serve to show how all the rest which perished at that time might have been preserved in their beneficence to the present day.

Newark College, Leicester (p. 29) was founded by the powerful family of Lancaster in the fourteenth century. At the Dissolution, its highly ecclesiastical portion disappeared, but its hospital, intended for 100 poor men, remains to this day. So do St. Ursula's, founded in Henry VI.'s time, and Wiggeston's, actually established in Henry VIII.'s early days, both in the same town of Leicester. It is not improbable that the protection of the Duchy of Lancaster caused preservation of these three hospitals.

Knolles' Hospital, Pontefract, founded by a layman of that name, was an almshouse attached to a college. The college was dissolved, but the almshouse was placed by Elizabeth under the Corporation, and remains. St. Giles', Norwich, was very ecclesiastically constituted. The monastic part was dissolved in the time of Edward VI., and the hospital placed under the Corporation of the city.

It is possible that several more hospitals which have survived had their ecclesiastical element removed without destruction of their charitable portion, but the data collected by the present writer do not reveal what exactly happened.

Survival.—It would be interesting to enquire the causes which enabled other hospitals to weather the storm. *A priori*, we might say that a lay foundation and a constitution, in which monasticism played but small part, preserved them. To a considerable extent this is true, yet some of the hospitals of this character fell, while some which were practically chantries, survived.

Lambourn, in Berkshire, seems to have been entirely lay, and was secured by an Act of Parliament in Elizabeth's reign. St. Bartholomew's, Oxford, had a royal foundation, a master, two " healthful " brethren (probably clerical), and six infirm. It was placed under Oriel College, which had to maintain it. Ewelme (Chap. VIII.) had a distinctly chantry element, but remained untouched, its carefully arranged constitution and maintenance in private hands securing it from destruction. Harbledown and St. John's, Canterbury, though ecclesiastically founded and probably monastic in constitution, survive, the power of the archbishops and good management in all likelihood saving them. St. Bartholomew's, Smithfield, and St. Thomas', Southwark, had clerical founders and clerical constitutions, and we know their history.

Some hospitals were, perhaps, too small and too *unprofitable* to invite dissolution, such as St. Margaret's, Wimborne, which was also in private hands, and Ely Davies' in Croydon. The influence of the queens probably preserved St. Katharine's, by the Tower of London, while St. Cross would receive the efficient support of the Bishops of Winchester.

On the other hand, among hospitals of lay foundation,

the great primal one established by King Athelstane was practically annihilated by Henry's commissioners in spite of its constitution being more lay than ecclesiastical. Those founded at Warwick by two different earls have disappeared ; Earl Arundel's has vanished ; of that at Sevenoaks, augmented by a layman in the fifteenth century, only the school remains ; Trinity at Dartford, though a corporation and of lay institution, was dissolved ; St. Mary's Spital in London, afterwards the New Hospital of our Lady, founded by lay people and providing for 180 *sick*, was nevertheless destroyed, and Elsing's, also in London, opened by a layman for 100 *blind men*, entirely ceased its benevolent intent. We may add to the list the late pre-Reformation hospital at Coventry.   The only dangerous provision of Ford was praying for his soul, but this led to its eventual suppression under an act of Edward VI. against chantries.

Number 13.—There are some further points of interest as throwing light on mediæval thought and custom. The number of thirteen is one of these, and it has already received comment.   That was the prescribed number as early as 1136 at St. Cross, as late as 1571 at Earl Leicester's hospital in Warwick, initially at Whitgift's in 1599, and we see it often in the intervening centuries. Yet Lanfranc, as early as 1085, provided for 100, Newark College in the fourteenth century for a like number.   Queen Maud's in the twelfth for 40 lepers, and at Sherburn, Durham, there was provision towards the end of the same century for 65, though these were divided into five " convents " of thirteen each, while we know that King Athelstane's hospital, the first of all, grew to vast proportions in the fourteenth century.

On the other hand, we have seen that some received quite a small number of inmates.

Survivals and Ceasings of Customs.—Nearly all mediæval hospitals were dedicated to some object of veneration—generally a patron saint. Saint John the Baptist, as a wanderer, stood pre-eminent, the reception of pilgrims entering largely into the objects of earlier hospitals, while St. John the Evangelist lagged far behind him. St. James received honour as being the patron at Compostella, the chief continental shrine. The name of Thomas à Beckett became popular after his " martyrdom " at Canterbury, while not a single hospital seems to have been built in honour of St. Thomas the Apostle, as if the Church had " no use " for doubters. St. Nicholas was often a patron, while St. Bartholomew is not infrequently named. St. Giles (Latinised, Egidius) was accounted patron saint of lepers (see p. 11), but St. Lazarus, who gave his name to lazar-houses, is only once mentioned in these pages as a patron. Divine dedications, *i.e.* to the Holy Saviour or the Holy Trinity, as distinct from saintly, were less frequent. Sacred objects or events appear in veneration of the Holy Cross and the Annunciation. St. Mary in some cases means the Mother of Christ, in others Mary Magdalene, who may have been chosen for hospitals specially, not because she was the first to speak with the risen Saviour, but because seven devils had been cast out of her by Christ.

Rare consecrations appear to the Angels Gabriel and Michael, and to the Saints Andrew, Anthony, Clement, Edmund, Helen, Julian, Paul and Peter. Dedication to saints and sacred objects ceased at the Reformation, while dedication in any form is entirely absent from Charter House and Sackville College, East Grinstead.

We have only noticed Incorporation at Ewelme and Dartford, but the survival of some hospital seals points to a wide extension of the practice if not the universal custom in mediæval times. The post-Reformation hospitals of Croydon and Guildford were corporations of the brethren (not the sisters) with the warden and master respectively, and the schoolmaster at the former, while the governors alone constituted a corporation at Charter House. Though this might be called a survival, it was needful when the protection—afterwards the bane—of the abbeys and priories was removed.

Mediæval insistence on attendance at the offices of the Church and praying for the souls of the dead benefactors survives, in an attenuated form, in the later hospitals. There we find the presence at daily prayers required, returning thanks for founders and benefactors, and going to church—in procession at Guildford, to an allotted chapel at Croydon. Likewise is the wearing of gowns at Guildford and Charter House—discontinued at Croydon—a mediæval survival.

The singleness of inmates enforced at Charter House and Guildford, a rule laid down by Whitgift but relaxed, is distinctly another monastic survival. It is curious that Ford's Hospital, founded 70 years before Whitgift's, did (at a little later date) provide for married couples, and that the little hospital at Wimborne has now three married among its nine inmates, though in this case it is not certain if it was the original intent of the founder.

So far as the writer knows, daily dining in hall only survives at Charter House, where it is clearly a continuation of the ancient practice usual in the monastic Refectory, honoured elsewhere only on " Gaudy Days " and such-like. Yet the common hall is a link with the remote past. The communal life is a precious legacy from that past conventual life (*con*, together, *venio*, *ventum*, come), when Benedict supplanted hermitage, which happily we have not altogether changed, and would like to see amplified.

Lastly, the silver thread—should we not rather say the golden ?—remains.

INDEX

Dedications, 143–4, 191–2.
Dorset, Earls of, 56–7.
Dress, 83, 128–9, 144, 148, 192.
Dowcra, Ld. Prior, 154.

Eadmer, 6, 82.
East India Comp., 94, 96.
Edmund, St. (King), Borough of, 80.
„ St. (Bishop), gilt cap of, 77.
Erasmus, 10.
Essex, county of, 85.
Evelyn, John, 96.
Ewelme, village of, 71.

Fishmongers' Comp., 67, 127.
Flagellation, 162–3.
Flambard, 21–2.
Fynche, Samuel, vicar and governor at Croydon, 93, 97–100, 113, 124–6.

Gaunt, John of, 29, 50–1, 166.
Giles, St., 11.
Gower, poet, 176.
Gray (of Elegy), 67.
Gresham, Ld. Mayor, 155, 160.
Gruesome effigies, 72–3 and footnotes.
Guest House, Audience, Guest, Great Chamber, 4, 140, 143, 146, 181.

Hampden, John, 67.
"Harbour of Refuge" (painting), 67.
Hartwell, Abraham, 93, 95, 113.
Harūn, Caliph, 5.
Herbert de Lozinga, 80.
Houghton, prior of Charter House, 168.
Howard of Effingham, 66.
Hospitium, 2.
Hospitals: Early Christian, 3, 4; Greek and Egyptian (temples), 3; Roman, 3; First in England, see York under **Hospitals.**
HOSPITALS TOPOGRAPHICALLY ARRANGED:
Abingdon, Christ's, formerly St. Helen's, 62–4.
Arundel, 56.
Banbury, St. John, 32.
Basingstoke, Walter de Merton's, 42–3.
Bath, St. John and Hosp. for lunatics, 39–40.
Bedford, St. John, St. Leonard, 34.
Bentley, Derbysh., Mount Joy's, 28–9.
Bethlehem, see **Insanity.**
Beverley, St. Giles, 19.
Bray, Jesus, 67.
Bridgewater, St. John, 40.
Bristol, St. Bart., Lyon's, Foster's, Barstaple's, 39.

HOSPITALS TOPOGRAPHICALLY ARRANGED (contd.):
Brough, W'morland, Sts. Mary and Gabriel, 20.
Bury St. Edmund's, St. John, St. Nicholas, St. Peter, St. Petronella, St. Saviour, St. Stephen, 80–81.
Canterbury, St. John, St. Gregory, 82–3.
Chichester, St. Mary, 55–6.
Cirencester, St. John, St. Leonard, 38.
Colchester, St. Mary Mag., 86.
Coventry, Ford's, Bablake, St. John, 24–6.
Croydon, Ely Davy's, 137, 189.
„ Whitgift's, see W.'s H. p. 199.
Doncaster, St. James, St. M. Mag., St. Nicholas, 18.
Dartford, Kent, Holy Trinity, 84.
Dover, St. Mary, 84.
Donnington, Berks, Atterbury's, 65
East Grinstead, Sackville Coll., 56–7.
East Hendred, Berks, 64.
Ewelme, Chap. VIII.
Exeter, Wynard's, Bonville's, St. Kath., Sts. Alexius and John, 35–6.
Gateshead, St. Edmund, 22.
Gloucester, St. Margaret, St. M. Mag., St. Bart., 38.
Glastonbury, Women's Almshouses, St. John, 40.
Guildford, St. Thos. (extinct), 137; Blessed Trinity (Abbot's), 136–150; contrasted with Whitgift's, 142–150.
Higham Ferrers, Northants, 31–2.
High Wycombe, St. John, 67–8.
Hereford, Conningsby's, St. Ethelbert, 28.
Hull, Kingston-upon-, Maison Dieu, Earl Suffolk's, 19.
Hythe, Kent, St. Andrew, 83–4.
Ilford, St. Mary, St. Thos., 86.
King's Lynn, St. Mary Mag., 76.
Kepier, Durham, St. Giles, 21.
Lambourne, Berks, Isbery's, 62.
Lewes, St. Jas., St. Nicholas, 56.
Lincoln, extinct lazar-houses, 76.
Leicester, Newark Coll., St. Ursula, Wiggeston's, 29.
Lutterworth, St. John, 30.
London: St. Anthony, 153–4; St. Bart., 159–60; St. Giles, 155; St. Kath. by Tower, 155; St. Mary of Beth., 160–1; St. Mary Spital, 157; St. Mary Overy, united with St. Thos.

O

For Product Safety Concerns and Information please contact our EU
representative GPSR@taylorandfrancis.com
Taylor & Francis Verlag GmbH, Kaufingerstraße 24, 80331 München, Germany

www.ingramcontent.com/pod-product-compliance
Lightning Source LLC
Chambersburg PA
CBHW070358270326
41926CB00014B/2604

9 7 8 0 4 1 5 8 2 1 4 5 2